Dear Babies

Crazy Life, Simply Explained

A<small>MY</small> D<small>ENBY</small>

ISBN: 1501074288
ISBN 13: 9781501074288
Library of Congress Control Number: 2014916262
CreateSpace Independent Publishing Platform
North Charleston, South Carolina

"And trustful birds have built their nests amid
The shuddering boughs, and only wait to sing."
—Robert Seymour Bridges

An Introduction:

Hello, My Name is Amy

Thursday, August 4, 2011

Dear Babies,

It is 4:15 PM on a steaming hot Thursday and I emerge from the train angry, as usual. It's what happens when an otherwise pleasant-enough woman arrives in Penn Station and finds herself thrust into the chaos of mad-dashing commuters. I have bags. I am sweating. I have to pee, but there is no stopping. A short pause and I would become swept up in the encroaching horde of aggressive men running to catch the 4:22 home to Long Island. I am walking against the grain, pushing up against a sea of scurrying people. Where is the once-upon-a-time glamour of Grand Central? The civilized men glancing casually at wrist watches in trench coats? Martinis in little glasses? Don Draper? Someone's luggage jabs me in the ribs.

—Ow-wah, that hurt!—

Obviously, not here.

I race up to 34th Street, skipping every other step in a soaring salute to my never-ending quest to lose baby weight. Or what I'd like to pretend is baby weight. The truth is, the bat wings and cellulite have always been there, but since living through the mind-boggling experience of a twin pregnancy, looking like I'd swallowed not just a basketball but a basketball team, I now chalk up any unsightliness to you, my two healthy, beautiful babies who at birth nine months ago weighed close to seven pounds each, rather than the fact that I'm a woman in my thirties who eats cheese. (It's the perfect alibi.) One day I hope to get to the point when I'll receive a compliment without a clause—"You look great! For just having had babies. . ." Until then, stairs.

It's sweltering.

I walk up 7th Avenue with my head held high, trying to convey coolness. Like, *I am not a tourist.* Like, *I used to live here. I lived in Soho! Tribeca! I used to buy my bananas with Eric Nies! But alas, it's useless. I cross the intersection toward Macy's with the rest of the commuters like the suburban stay-at-home mom that I am. The driver of a three-row-car with a short hairdo whose idea of a "crazy night" means staying up until eleven to watch the latest franchise of Real Housewives. And let's face it, nobody cares about Eric Nies. Who, you ask? Exactly.*

No one knows about my former life. How I used to walk through Washington Square Park on my way to work early in the morning. How alive it could feel even when empty, especially in the fall. There's my bench, *I'd think. I also had a tree. And a buddy, a bearded homeless man who held up a sign everyday scrawled with different funny sayings, like* "Need money for beer so I can get girls drunk and have a threesome." *I was part of the New York heartbeat. A writer who lived on Thompson Street. My heels clacked on the pavement up West Fourth Street, keeping the pulse—*

Watch it! *a voice yells.*

A car slams on its horn.

I am on 35th Street now, and those days are gone.

"Where are you?" your father says on the other end of the phone. No hello.

"I'm here, where are you?"

"Around the corner."

Delighted, I end the call and wipe the screen, now sticky with moisturizer and perspiration, before slipping it into my overstuffed bag. I beat him.

"Ha, ha!" I taunt as I see your father approaching. He crosses in front of a bead and fabric shop advertising bedazzled Quinceanera dresses on sale for $14.99. He's sweating, poor guy. Still, I beat him, a fact that should not go unnoticed. "You thought I was going to be late!"

We kiss, mixing our summer-in-the-city lip sweat.

"I did." I am always late. But he has "the Mike face" on. The serious face. The can-you-not-be-a-child-for-like-two-minutes face. "Let's go," he says, not in the mood for banter. He holds open the old door of the building and, quiet, we proceed inside, then step into a rickety elevator.

I look down at my feet. At my dirty, unpolished shrimp-cocktail toes. I need a pedicure. A manicure. A haircut. An eyebrow wax. I need to take a shower without one eye on a baby monitor across the room through the steam. (It would be nice to have the time to shave my legs with shaving cream. Maybe even do above the knee.)

I've never been to see a lawyer before.

The office is surprisingly modern, at least compared to the outdated lobby downstairs.

Schma-la-la, Ra-la-la, Visk-kish-la-la, and Smith, or something like that.

Inside, there are so many books.

Sooooo many books.

I wonder if the many hardcover books lining the walls are empty replicas, props like the ones I used to rent when I was a producer for photo shoots at J.Crew, those fall shoots that always required "scholarly" touches like apples and trophies and Lauren Hutton in black rimmed glasses. Your dad is preoccupied by his Blackberry. I am tempted to pick up the Wall

Street Journal in front of me and quote Romy and Michele's
High School Reunion—do you have some sort of biz-ness
woman special?—*but I don't. Instead, I nudge your father to
stop scrolling. This is not the place for work or monkey business. We're here to sign our wills in case, God forbid, heaven
forbid, no, no, please God, NO! forbid, something happens to
us, your parents.*

"Mike!" *A man in a blue collared shirt and black slacks
emerges from a glass-enclosed conference room. He extends
a well-manicured bear paw.* "Nice to see you!" *They heartily
shake. He looks like a lawyer. At least, I think he does. I don't
really get lawyers; I don't know why they have to talk like that,
why adding a* "th" *to the end of a word makes it sound* "legal."
It's dumb and yet, still intimidating. "Whereath." *Is that even
a word? But I suppose if you were in need of a lawyer, you'd
want this guy to be in your corner. Big. Strong. Like bull.*

Inside the fishbowl we quickly get down to business.

*Stacks of one-inch-thick documents get slid across the
table. But pens. Where are the pens? Our lawyer stalks off,
out into the hall, where he grumbles to no one in particu-
lar about how everyone takes the pens from the conference
room. I watch him through the glass as he moves from desk
to desk—do they really all work in these dingy cubicles?
They're all smart, they say whereath, shouldn't they have
nicer offices? He comes back with three good ones. Click,
click, click. Thick rubber grips. Silky black ink. Check my
pockets on the way out, sir, because I would steal these in a
heartbeat.*

*The first order of business is setting up the trust. I can't
imagine what it would be like if we were millionaires because,*

trust me (nudge, nudge), this is a pretty complicated thing even when you're not.

"So say they're gamblers, right? You don't know, you don't KNOW! They can't touch anything until they're thirty-five. Okay, twenty-five. Thirty. And then thirty-five, they get the rest. You do this in increments because," and he stresses his point by making eye contact with us individually, one after the other, "you don't know." This is before he proceeds to talk about all the financial stuff and estates taxes and things that go completely over my head and cause my eyes to glaze over.

"Right," your dad says when the lawyer finally finishes, and he means it. He understands this. He has his pen in hand and he's ready to sign.

I am wide-eyed like I Love Lucy.

Tumbleweeds would be blowing through my mind if they weren't so knotted and confused.

"Any questions?" the lawyer asks politely.

There is a sizable pause, during which maybe I blink, overwhelmed, before he drops his head and turns to the next page in the massive document. Moving on.

"Let's hope they're not gamblers!" The words fling themselves out of my mouth like lemmings throwing their bodies off the edge of a cliff.

"I'm sorry?" he says, as if I'd just spoken in Chinese.

Your father sneaks me a sympathetic grin.

I swallow my words, a weak attempt at humor to diffuse my unease, and then we do move on.

What strikes me as so odd about the whole will-signing is how casually our lawyer handles it.

"So say you have a family disaster, okay? Something happens to the four of you, you all die—"

"OKAY!" I want to shout. "I GET IT! WE DIE! GAME OVER! FINITO! But do you really have to say it?"

But yes, he has to say it, because that's what we're here for. To not just say it, but to say it in front of witnesses and get it notarized. To write it down. To make it legal. Whereath. I am going to die, and if God-forbid I do die before I get to wear muumuus down in Florida like the Golden Girls, then I have to plan for who will take care of you.

And it sucks.

But I don't have a choice.

I am an adult.

A mother.

You think it would be strangely comforting, this affirmation that it really does matter if my existence gets wiped from the planet—who will take care of you?!—but it's not.

I sit silently, staring down at the black ink on the pages and pages before me. I'm not seeing anything, just a blur, of roman numerals, some names in all caps, dotted lines for signatures. I am lost in thought. How can the most universal symbol of life—you guys, my babies! The best thing in the whole wide world!—have landed me here, face to face with my own mortality?

"Say something happens to Mike, okay? Then Amy, you and your sister have to. . . " *and he goes on and on and on about how to access accounts and write checks and good lord.*

And my heart clenches with pangs of sadness at the possibility.

"Say something happens to Amy. . ."

"You alright?" your dad asks an hour later as we descend in the same rickety elevator.

"Yeah, that was just a lot. . ."

"It was a lot. . ."

"Yeah, it was. . . a lot."

A lot. How moments of great impact sometimes translate into the littlest words.

"Subway? Taxi?" I ask casually once we get to the corner. We're headed downtown for dinner—the new date night, dinner and a will-signing. I'm hoping he says taxi. I want to see the city. See the streets. See the lights. Pass restaurants and recognize landmarks and feel comforted that they're still there, like I am still a part of it all. "My coffee place!" "I ate lunch there after I bought my wedding dress!" "Gobo! We used to get take-out from there all the time!"

I am looking forward to dinner, and when I say dinner I mean a big, fat goblet-sized refreshing glass of wine that they always seem to be drinking on those Real Housewives shows before throwing them in people's faces. I want to shake the heaviness of the afternoon off and enjoy this night out with your dad. I have to. These days, they are few and far between. And look, I am here! I am back in the city! I have a babysitter and I am downtown! I have to put these serious thoughts and crazy fears of impending doom out of my head. What if, what if?!

"What if we went someplace down by the West Village?"

"Okay."

We park ourselves in the corner of a dark wine bar on Bleecker Street that enticed us with its flickering candles and funky reggae music. In the dim light I can make out a stuffed wild boar hanging from a white subway-tiled wall, how anything goes with these places. Boars Head Bologna meets Parisian bathroom, ah, this must be the new thing! Though I'll admit, the glassy finish of the tiles reflects all the *candlelight nicely and gives the whole room a warm, orange glow. At high tables nearby couples huddle together over plates of olives and cured meats. I order a glass of Soave. Cold, crisp, delicious. For your father, pinot noir. And then the bar top buzzes. Your dad's Blackberry is going off.*

Damn.

"I'm sorry, babe, there's all this drama. . ."

"I know," I say. And I do.

Your father spends the rest of the evening hunched over his phone, frantically typing away with his thumbs while I am left to fend off creeping thoughts, like nothing goes as imagined. . .

I begin to feel like I am not even there.

I drink. . .

I people watch. . .

The manager, with his white shirt unbuttoned and shaggy hair long, chases a girl out the door.

"Hey, hey!" he calls, running after her when she rises from her barstool and takes one last sip of her pink champagne. "What's your name?"

"Ali," I hear her answer.

He is Marc.

I watch them talk on bustling Bleecker Street through the open window. They smile. She touches his arm. I see her point somewhere. Where?

"I live just around the corner. . ." I imagine she says.

Did her invite her to a party?

Or to his other more intimate—no, hipper—restaurant around the block where he will meet her later tonight?

Beside them a couple embraces. She in a striped dress. He, slim jeans. Both of them so young. What do they know? What could they know? He touches her thigh in a place that would cause me, at my age with my cellulite, to shy away.

And then the couple walks in.

They take a seat across from each other at a table nestled in the back.

I take another sip. I begin a game with myself, what would I say if seated across from a stranger right now?

(Oh, the stories I could tell.)

Where on earth would I begin?

Hello, my name is Amy, though that's not the only name I answer to.

I spend most of my time with my now toddler twins who only know me by a different name, a one-word moniker so bold it stands on its own. I am kind of like Madonna (but not really). I am Mom.

What's great about being Mom, besides having my own section in the greeting card aisle and access to a constant graze of Pepperidge Farm Goldfish to boot, is living in the presence of tangible hope. Children are little clean slates of promise. Maybe they'll be smarter than you. Maybe they'll be kinder than you. Maybe they'll have it better than you. Maybe they will be the ones who make the world a better place.

Each day mine blow me away. No, I mean they actually blow me away like the Big Bad Wolf huffing and puffing and I am the meek little pig, outnumbered (twin toddlers!).

I write daily letters to them like the one you just read about this funny life of ours, because I'm a writer, and that's what I do. I don't tell them how to do things. I am a far cry from Emily Post. I have a piece of paper from Penn State University that says I am a journalist, so I guess I am that. I journal. I observe. I tell them how life is. I tell them about little things, like how I bring back giant packs of toilet paper from Costco and hoard them in our basement like an ant. I tell them about big things, like war, how it stinks and I can't fix it (but maybe they can?). I reflect on my growing pains, thinking *maybe I can stop them from doing one of the myriad stupid things that I have done*, from streaking my hair with Jolen mustache bleach to putting a marshmallow in the microwave—all the while realizing the importance of those bumps. That they, too, will have to learn how to fall (though preferably not for Brazilian DJ's). After all (spoiler alert), I am a parent who has no idea what I'm doing. All I really want is to keep them safe, and alive. And if I can do that while they become yellow-haired-candy-torching-pyros, I'll take it . . . though I kind of wish I didn't just put that in writing.

Recently I wrote to them, "It's hard to see yourself the way others see you." This pearl of wisdom arose regarding my husband, their father, commenting that I look like Kurt from *Glee*. But whatever, it got me thinking about this person, Amy, and how she saw herself over the years.

Growing up in the late-eighties in Long Island, I longed to be Cindy Mancini in *Can't Buy Me Love* with that white-suede fringe outfit. *Like, oh my God!*, I would say, banishing my Fran Drescher roots and trying to talk like the gum-smacking Valley Girls so popular at the time. I was going to marry Jordan Knight from the New Kids on the Block and write books like the Nancy Drew series. Then, as a teenager in the nineties, I kept my thing for brown-eyed boys but decided I was going to marry Freddie Prinze Junior instead. A teen sleuth series changed to fashion articles for *Vogue*. In college, *Sex and the City* came out. I met Carrie Bradshaw and was like, hallelujah!, now *that* is going to be me. I was going to be single and fabulous when I graduated, having adventures with my girlfriends while looking for Mr. Big in NYC. I started wearing a big flower pin like Carrie around campus. Once a frat boy asked me if I was a clown, as if I was going to squirt him with water.

The truth is. . .

With braces and a whopping case of insecurity, I was the opposite of Cindy Mancini.

Freddie Prinze Junior married Buffy the Vampire Slayer.

I did grow up to write for a few magazines, but never for *Vogue*.

And I was single for about five minutes after graduation. I met my husband, and we've been together ever since. We had adventures in New York City. And he has the brightest blue eyes you have ever seen.

Amy saw life going one way.

Mom knows that life likes to go the other.

My husband, Mike, and I are soul mates, the kind that honestly tell each other when the other smells like onions, the kind that miss each other when the other leaves the room.

We enjoyed a long engagement. We traveled. We slept in seaside cottages along the Cote d'Azur. In January of 2008 we had a dream wedding overlooking Central Park on a clear winter's night. That May we "pulled the goalie," as our financial adviser so eloquently phrased our decision to go off birth control. Here's where you say 1.) We sound very annoying, and 2.) We have a very involved financial guy. But my point in telling you this is. . . we were young. We were healthy. We were excited. We talked about putting up a wall in our one bedroom apartment to make room for the baby. We bought packs of drug store home pregnancy tests. I imagined myself taking one while my husband was at work. I knew exactly how I would tell him our good news. . .

We never saw ourselves as a couple who wouldn't be able to get pregnant.

After about six months of irregular menstrual cycles—and no babies—I found myself snowballing down a road of doctor's appointments and blood tests and bad news that lasted two years. Each visit went kind of like this: *"Wait, what? I have to do what this time around? What is that? And how much is this going to cost?"* Before I knew it, my fridge was stocked with enough vials of fertility medication and syringes to turn my prewar kitchen in the Upper West Side into a French County methadone lab.

One of the many crazy things about undergoing fertility treatments is how you reach a point where it all becomes normal. When you first learn you have to give yourself daily injections you think you're never going to be able to do it. Then, you're giving yourself four shots a night in your thigh like it is *nothing,* casually huffing "these idiots" under your breath while watching *Jersey Shore.* You don't even notice when you start making smarmy jokes throughout the internal sonograms, which during treatment might happen daily for weeks, quipping to a strange man in scrubs between your thighs—*"Oh, I have a lot of eggs on both ovaries? (nudge, nudge) Well, why put all of my eggs in one basket!"*

There are things you never get used to, of course. The cyclic hope and disappointment. The feeling like everyone else in the entire world is pregnant. Even Pam from *The Office.* (Come on!) The trying to figure out what you did to deserve this. Why you are being punished. Why you can't just have sex and get pregnant like, oh, I don't know, *the rest of the human race.* The choking back tears when another friend announces she's "preggo." (You're happy for her, sure, but it's hard. And how annoying is the word preggo?) You never get used to people—from older relatives to chirpy co-workers—seeing you without child and offering their unsolicited advice. *Relax! Don't think about it! The minute I stopped thinking about it, I got pregnant! Have sex every other day! Use the rhythm method! Just look for your fertile mucus! Go home, have a glass of wine and have fun with your husband {wink}!* You find yourself wanting to punch all of these people in the face. And you never saw yourself as a violent person. And that's a lot of people you want to punch in the face.

I know torture.

I know I exaggerate (see above, "writer").

I know a lot of people know real torture, in various capacities, but torture for me is a two-week wait time after you just spent $14,000 on an IVF cycle you were told didn't go so well.

You can't take a pregnancy test because with all of the hormones you've been on, the results would be false. You can't exercise or do yoga or take a bath. You can't sleep. After a three-day pity party to the soundtrack from *La Vie En Rose*, you can't listen to music anymore. Or phone commercials. You can't even (horror of horrors) drink.

Then, suddenly, you don't feel well. Granted, you haven't felt well for a while—during an average menstrual cycle a woman experiences cramps and bloating while producing one egg; after six weeks of multiple hormone injections, you had produced 29—but this *feels* different. Yet, you don't want to let yourself think you might be pregnant. You can't, and your husband won't let you. He's afraid you won't be able to recover again. (He's afraid he can no longer wear the mask of strength.) It could be your body coming off all the drugs, *but it could be morning sickness...*

On day fourteen you go in for a pregnancy blood test and you spend the rest of the morning trying to run from your mind, wandering the streets of New York City beside your husband, speechless, like two jellyfish. You spend hours in the Apple Store. You come home and watch *The Blind Side* and right before you're about to find out what college the kid got into, the phone rings—

Amy? Congratulations, you're pregnant.

And the next adventure begins...

What follows on these pages are the letters I wrote to our babies throughout my pregnancy.

They are my life. My air. My reason for seeing the world as a brighter place. My reason for seeing it as so goddamn scary.

They blow me away. And no, I don't mean in the Big Bad Wolf-sense huffing and puffing. I mean they awe-inspiringly, heart-achingly, I could sit here for hours watching them, stealing kisses on their tiny limbs, blow me away.

When I first found out I was pregnant, I called my mom. Then, I opened my laptop and began to write. After all, I was supposed to be Carrie Bradshaw.

For anyone who wants to know what it's really like to be pregnant. For anyone who knows and wants a fresh outlook on parenting's ups and downs. For anyone seeking inspirations. For anyone at a crossroad, surrendering to change...

Dear Babies,
This is crazy life, simply explained. . .

POPPY SEEDS.

Thursday, March 11, 2010

Dear Babies,

I just found out yesterday that you are here and already I love you so much I feel as if my heart might burst. (Or, that could be heartburn.) Your father and I, we just cried so much. . .

When I wasn't sure if you were going to make it to our first pregnancy blood test I went ahead and told you about all the crazy, wonderful people in our family you could get to meet if you stayed, *remember*? I told you about my mom, your grandma, the nicest, most loving, damn-near angelic person in the world. She has these bright blue eyes and adorable, freckled, pink Irish cheeks. She's been praying and lighting so many candles for you I'm sure Christ the Church in Long Island is visible right now from space. After we got the phone call I called and told her the news. She, too, burst into tears, and cried, "Mickey, Mickey! They're pregnant!" So, dear babies, after the doctor, after your father and I, after your grandma, the next recipient of the joyous news that at least one of two embryos we had implanted two weeks ago through in-vitro fertilization took was an obese chocolate lab named Mickey. The dog looks like a coffee table. He loves nothing more than to sleep all day sprawled out on a plush wraparound couch in central air conditioning and watch soap operas. I told you that your grandma was a really good cook, and how she will love to feed you. How she loves to feed everyone, baked ziti, meatballs, lasagna, or my favorite, her eggplant parmesan. She's such a good cook. (Don't worry, she learned from your grandpa's side, the Italians; you don't want the Irish side to make anything except reservations.) She wants to be called Nanny. That's what her mother was called.

I told you about Aunt Krissy, my older sister whom I tease mercilessly but deep-down secretly idolize, always have, always will. She is equally excited and decided that she wants to be called "Auntie" Krissy, aunt being too formal. She went to our parents' house and with your Nanny and our dad—who said he wants to be called "Boompah" instead of Grandpa, and we'll just leave that at that— toasted with Doritos and champagne.

Your other grandma, your dad's mom, is Mimi. I told you she was really pretty and a lot of fun and that she was really good at making people feel better. She's from Texas. There's an expression people say that goes, "everything is bigger in Texas." I can say this is especially true when it comes to the size of their hearts. When Mimi sees you getting upset she'll think nothing of throwing her arms around you and sweeping you up into a dance and away from your troubles. She's right, by the way. Life is better when you dance. True to her reputation as the life of the party, last night she hopped in a car from Queens and surprised us with a knock on the door, just to hug us, just to share our tears of joy, and of course have some sips of champagne. . .

Your Aunt Michele (Shelly for short), your dad's sister, was also there to celebrate. If you're a girl then I hope you're like either of your two aunts, or an amazing hybrid of them both. Aunt Shelly is very upset that we don't want to find out your sex until the day you're born and you can show us yourselves. In fact she's already plotting ways to pry the coveted information from our doctor, and probably shopping for a new trench coat and sunglasses to wear for that occasion as we speak.

But, for now, we don't care about your sex.

We don't care about little pink dresses.

A nursery of sailboats in red, white and blue.

Even your names.

(Though, I'm not gonna lie, we already started making jokes about "Dick Denby," it's quite possibly the best name ever.)

Right now we just care about you, and that you continue to grow into strong and healthy babies. That you get everything you need from us, all of our love and support. That you stay with us.

Please, babies, stay, *stay*. . .

We go in for our second blood test tomorrow.

I love you.

Love,
Mom

Friday, March 12, 2010

Dear Babies,

Our hcg level doubled, whoo-hoo! Today we're up to 462. Yesterday was a treat having a nurse speak simple English on the phone—*congratulations, you're pregnant*—as opposed to a biology-heavy conversation on drug dosages and hormone levels and the number of follicles on my left ovary. *The usual.* Things that most people do not know about, that you should probably never know about, but that I know about after my two year stint as the human pin cushion. Today, back to bio, we spoke of the results of the blood test measuring my level of *human chorionic gonadotropin*, "the pregnancy hormone." I Google. I know 462 is a high hcg number for this stage, four weeks pregnant. I know this is good.

Yet, I'm so nervous I can barely breath.

I'm scared something's going to happen. I'm afraid to move. I'm afraid of bleeding. I don't want to lose you. I sit paralyzed the days of these blood tests, wide-eyed and mute like a rabbit. I don't want the doctor to call and deliver the news that would take this all away.

Ah, dammit. Why did I go on that Web site and read all about the signs of early pregnancy miscarriages?

Stay away from the Internet, use it only to buy things you don't need. (See my assortment of shawls.)

I spoke to a nurse three hours ago and she told me that everything was fine. So why am I being crazy?

{Inhale, exhale.}

Shake it off.

Just breathe, just be, let God, let go. . .

Everything is fine. You're still here. Your father says he knows its twins, *"if they put two in during our implantation. . .*" He's the logical one. I'm the gypsy who does not want to jinx things. I think its twins, too, but I'll never admit it. Not until our first ultrasound when it can physically be confirmed. I know I can't let myself think these good things yet. I know I can't get too excited. I know I can't get my hopes up, but. . .

You're both growing. You're both healthy and strong. I can feel it.

This is my turn.

Love,
Mom

Monday, March 15, 2010

Dear Babies,

Your dad called just now to tell me that he is related to the King of Scotland, King James Stewart the IV. He's been obsessed with ancestry.com ever since he saw that show a few weeks ago on NBC where celebrities track down their ancestors. Sarah Jessica Parker went all the way back to the Salem Witch trials, when one of her ancestors was charged as a witch. Maybe you'll watch her in *Sex and the City* reruns with me someday, or *Footloose* out in 1984. You'll probably cringe and say, 'this movie is so old,' like when my parents used to show me their favorites when I was little—Shirley Temple tap-dancing to "On the Good Ship Lollipop"—and I'd roll my eyes and say just that, so *old*, like old was a disease. Like it went the dinosaurs, then my parents. But I promise, my old movies will be good. (*Or is that something all old people say?*)

Tonight I was supposed to have dinner with my girl-friends but it got cancelled. Which means that box of cute little St. Patrick's Day cookies I bought for my friend's adorable two-year-old son? Yup, all ours. In fact I'm biting the head off a jigging flame-haired leprechaun as we speak. Mmm, butter. I wonder, what *is* fondant?

By now I hope you're getting comfortable in your new home for the next nine months. (Meanwhile, a pregnancy is 40 weeks; divided by four weeks in a month, that's *ten* months. They must tell we pregnant gals nine for motivation. Doctors basically saying, *it's okay, tell a little white lie to keep them happy*.) I'm sorry it's not nicer, and it doesn't have any windows. But if it makes you feel any better the view from my window here on West 89th Street, a fire escape and three brick walls, isn't that great, either. I think your dad and I might move. Not now, though. Now we're still taking things one step at a time.

I followed a man for half a block today in the rain just to return the pen he'd dropped—he said thank you and walked on, what did I expect, a medal? And last week when I saw a homeless man rinsing his mouth out behind his junk-laden shopping cart with a water bottle filled with what I hoped was just dirty water, I gave him a dollar and a pack of gum. I thought, karma, you know? Maybe it will help keep you. . .

Third blood test tomorrow.

I'm so nervous I can't do a thing. Not move or breath or speak. I need to shake my head and stop thinking about it. I need to stop torturing myself with the what-ifs. I need to. . . go watch *The Bachelor.* Say what you will about reality television ("the dumbing down of America!" we say at dinner parties pretending to be smart, with hours of *Survivor* logged on our DVRs at home) but it's the perfect antidote for pregnancy. Mindless distraction? Yes, please.

Love,
Mom

SESAME SEEDS.

Tuesday, March 16, 2010

Dear Babies,

Our hcg level reached 2,056 today!!!! Yaaay!!! The nurse said this was a really good number! We were hoping to be around 1,000, the "magic number," I learned, we'd need to schedule our first ultrasound to see if you are both still here, if I am indeed having *twins*, and now we can!

Oh, babies, I'm so happy.

Each step I feel like we're getting closer, like it's—you're—becoming more real.

I got so nervous, as usual, this afternoon waiting for the phone call. That menstrual-like cramping I was feeling last week subsided and in not feeling anything I feared you were no longer here.

I know, I know, I have to calm down.

I should use my tiredness as reassurance. I've always heard pregnant friends complain of being *soooo tired*. And I would say something like *oh, that sucks* while quietly envying their state, thinking you stupid beotch, *I'd kill to be that tired.*

Well today I was so tired I contemplated resting my head on the shoulder of the man seated next to me on the subway. This wouldn't have been that crazy, the New York City transit system being the Mecca for crazies, the L train their Cheers where everybody knows their name.—"Hey, there's the preacher who looks like Meatloaf!"—but I'm not ready to go public as a pregnant lady yet.

I am however, ready to say no to green beer. Tomorrow is St. Patrick's Day. What a delight to pass on feeling my age at an Upper East Side bar, half-dancing to "Come on Eileen" while secretly looking for the exit signs fretting *it's a fire hazard in here.*

Instead I'll be home, looking up things I shouldn't be on the Internet for a change.

I Google-image searched "5 weeks pregnant." I'm not gonna lie, you look really weird. Kind of like alien slugs. The plant from Little Shop of Horrors meets Mr. Hanky. They say you're the size of a sesame seed, and that's a pretty small thing to be.

Love,
Mom

Wednesday, March 17, 2010

Dear Babies,

I just got back from a walk around the reservoir in Central Park. It's gorgeous out today. About 65 degrees. In case you work in a cubicle one day, happen to glance out the window and wonder, *who the heck are all of these people walking around the City in the middle of the afternoon?* I'll tell you: Beautiful people. So beautiful they apparently don't have to work. The park was *full* of such lookers in stylish running gear, sleek lululemon pants and black racerback tops—and me, dressed like Darby O'Gill in brown corduroy pants and an emerald green sweater vest. Because nothing says fitness like a leprechaun, *gees*. I had a plaid winter jacket tied around my waist, *and you can't really tie a winter jacket around your waist*. Let's consider this a rite of passage: First time you were embarrassed by something your mom wears.

As I walked up the east side of the runners path I could hear the bagpipers and drummers playing from the St. Patrick's Day parade on Fifth Avenue. I turned my music off—Paul Simon's *Graceland*, an album you'll love, it's like listening to summer—and listened to the revelry. With the sun shining on my face, my hair blowing lightly in the breeze, I felt like I was marching with them. Your great-grandparents, my grandparents, Nan and Poppy, were Irish. When I first found out I was pregnant with you I wished so badly that they were still alive so I could tell them, but then I felt better thinking that they were the ones who had answered my prayers up in heaven, that they already knew.

As I walked I passed a cluster of birds pecking at a sandwich bag with a crumbled muffin in it. The birds were trying so hard to get to the crumbs inside but they couldn't open the bag. I wanted to help them—*ninety-percent of birds are monogamous, you know, that says something of a species!*—I wanted to squat down and open it up for them, sprinkle out the crumbs and present them with a feast like I was the Barefoot Contessa and they were my feathered Jeffreys, *bon appetit!* But then, I thought, *nah,* germs. Plus I didn't feel like bending. So I kept walking.

But as I grew further away I began to panic, *what if they do get the bag open but then get stuck inside it and suffocate and die?* Because that's the best way to enjoy an afternoon stroll, berate yourself for a bird's hypothetical murder. *Why didn't I just open the bag for them?!* I thought maybe the birds would still be there on the loop back on my return, but no. They were gone. The bag remained intact, crumbled muffin inside preserved.

It could've been so good for them. . .

Life is full of little split second decisions like this one that may not appear to mean anything, babies, but sometimes I think mean everything. As Lucille Ball once said (and I do love Lucy!) (I know, *old*): "I would rather regret the things I've done than the things I haven't done."

Love,
Mom

Monday, March 22, 2010

Dear Babies,
    I lost a favorite sock in the wash today and it's really annoying.
    That's all.

Love,
Mom

LENTILS.

Thursday, March 25, 2010

Dear Babies,

Right when the ultrasound came on the screen yester-day I could clearly see two huge black blobs and all that I'd felt and hoped and prayed for came true:

"How do you feel about twins?," our doctor said with a smile.

I reached back while lying on the table and grabbed your father's hand. It was a magical moment, despite the fact that I was spread eagle and had a man on a stool be-tween my knees inserting an ultrasound wand where the sun don't shine. And we just started to cry, and we haven't stopped crying since, along with smiling stupidly at strang-ers, at trees, at unsuspecting mothers pushing double-wides down Broadway. *We have a secret, we are having twins!*

Babies, I feel so blessed. And yet still, so terrified.

Part of me feels like I don't deserve this. I'm scared if I'm happy and "let my guard down" I'm going to do some-thing to jinx this and make it all go away.

But, no, I must reassure myself, *that's not going to hap-pen.* I must think positive. I must!

The doctor heard two little heartbeats, already, at six weeks! You guys are the size of lentils! And they were *strong* heartbeats. They were too faint for us to hear but we could see them, pulsing away frantically on the screen.

You are now known medically as "Baby A" and "Baby B," two gray dots the doctor pointed out were good-size "yolk sacs" and "fetal poles," oh the intricate things we're learning about the human body so fast. I look at people in amazement now and wonder *how the heck are we all here?*

Your dad's aunt said this on the phone yesterday: *It's so hard to understand God's plan when you're in the thick of it and you can't understand why this is happening to you or why he is doing this to you, but then, just like that, there is a light at the end of the tunnel and everything does make sense. You just have to have faith. . .*

I have faith, babies, that everything is going to be all right.

I sang to you this morning in the shower, *don't worry, about a thing, cause every little thing is gonna be all right.* Bob Marley's "Three Little Birds." After all, there are three of us.

How bad of a singer am I, by the way?

And on another note, how good was that muenster cheese? I tell ya, there's nothing better than thinly sliced cheese that comes from the deli counter in folded wax paper.

I love you both.

Love,
Mom

Friday, March 26, 2010

Dear Babies,

I just licked a bowl of macaroni-and-cheese clean, scraping the hardened melted-cheese off the sides with fierce determination to get every last drop.

This is something I would've done before I was pregnant with you.

Just wanted to clear that up.

Love,
Mom

Monday, March 29, 2010

Dear Babies,

I feel like Matt Damon beefing up for a movie role. I'm supposed to drink a gallon of water a day, eat 90-140 grams of protein, 600 extra calories. If I gain the suggested weight for someone pregnant with twins, 45 pounds, this means I will soon weigh in at around 170 . . .

Babies, my whole life I was crazy and thought I was fat. I tried every fad exercise there is (you won't believe me when I tell you about the ThighMaster). I picked the cheese off of pizza. This is crazy because 1.) I was never fat, and 2.) Why would any sane person pick cheese off of pizza? That's the *point* of pizza. Cheese + tomato sauce+dough=*pizza*. I should've just eaten bread.

Now faced with legitimate weight that would've sent me running to the basement to do "Buns of Steel" (yes), I have to finally let go. Good-bye to the weight of my weight issues.

I'll be the happiest, while at my heaviest.

Whomever's pulling the strings up there, teaching us things, taking us down these twists and turns to get to the answers, must have a very wry sense of humor.

Love,
Mom

BLUEBERRIES.

Tuesday, April 6, 2010

Dear Babies,

In case you're wondering, air has a smell. Particularly cold air. I know this now because the scent of it suddenly makes me want to vomit. I run past grocery store doors to avoid such gusts of death.

Morning sickness can't be *real*, I once thought. *Of course you're going to feel like crap, you're pregnant!* Now, I look like Morgan Freeman with these broken capillaries around my eyes from barfing. Yes, I said barf.

I'm starving, yet can't eat anything, or rather can't keep anything down. (When there's nothing left to give I dry heave, that's my specialty. Olympic dry-heaving.)

People try to help. They tell me things. Don't eat and drink at the same time. The wet/dry method. Wait forty-five minutes after you eat to drink! Me and the Gremlins, *don't feed us after midnight.* "Here's a Preggo Pop," they say. To which I want to say, "I'm sorry, did I mention that air makes me want to vomit? *Do you know that air is every-where?*" And they think a *sucking candy* is going to help?

Apart from the slight daily misery, all is well, babies. We are seven weeks now. You guys are each the size of a blue-berry. Yes, everything is great.

We heard your two little heartbeats on Friday, thump-ing away like charging race horses. We didn't know what was happening when the doctor said, "okay, let's take a lis-ten," and then one, two, three he futzed around with some buttons on the ultrasound machine. I can never get over how these archaic-looking machines work such wonderful magic. They look like 1970s time machines. The next thing we knew *ka-thunk-ka-thunk-ka-thunk-ka-thunk* was filling the air. One of you already has a nickname, "the little guy," since you are measuring a few days behind the other in size but have the faster heartbeat. 156 beats-per-minute. "He's a little guy, but he's all heart," your dad remarked, like you're a scrappy prized boxer (like you're definitely a he). His big blue eyes were wide and glowing fixed on that screen.

These past two years weren't easy for your dad. He had to be strong for me. He had to swallow his fears. He had to take my hand and promise me everything was going to be all right, even when he didn't know if that was true. He couldn't take care of his wife. He couldn't start a family. Today, the goofy way he was smiling? That was happiness. I saw it with my own two eyes. I like to think that I am armed now. That whatever happens in life, when we're old sitting in our rockers, I will have the memory of this look.

Ooh God, I suddenly feel as if I am about to birth the tap-dancing alien from the end of *Spaceballs* from my chest.

Damn air.

Love,
Mom

KIDNEY BEANS.

Wednesday, April 7, 2010

Dear Babies,

"How does it feel having three kids?" your dad asked me teasingly as I opened my eyes first thing this morning.

I heard him come in last night around 1:30. I was awake in bed with my eyes closed, *Man vs. Food* or something like that flickering in the background. My head, the room spinning around me. *Sick, sick, so sick, must sleep, can't sleep.* I knew he was going to be home late tonight from his annual work party. I did not know that this year the party was at Lucky Strikes bowling alley, or that he'd be coming home in a bowling shirt like Johnny Nogerelli in *Grease 2*.

—*"Let's bowl, let's bowl, let's, rock and roll!"*—

. . . He's had some drinks.

He's flapping his gums.

He gets into bed next to me and won't stop talking, talking, *talking*. He stinks of stale beer and I roll over and try to ignore him. How do I feel. *Uhn.* That actress with the nose was there. *Uhn.* She seems like a total moron. *Uhhhn.* When he finally does shut up and fall asleep he starts snoring, loudly. I am married to Paul Bunyan. I elbow him, hard. He stops. He starts. I elbow him again. We begin a game of horizontal whack-a-mole.

Three hours later, I'm still sick, still exhausted, still can't sleep, *must sleep, must sleep, if only I could sleep!*, I hear a commotion like the Titanic crashing in our bathroom.

"Mike!" I yell, noticing that he's no longer by my side.

"Shh, babe, don't worry! It's just the ice," he hollers back.

"Oh, okay," I say as if this makes sense, delirious and rolling back over.

Silence.

Silence.

Then his words sink in and register. *"What??"*

"Don't worry, it's just the... ice..." and the commotion picks up again.

I haul myself out of bed like an out-of-shape superhero in a sports bra and giant grandma underwear. Your dad is in the bathroom hunched over a mop like Schneider from *One Day at a Time*, in his boxer shorts, amidst an insane amount of shattered glass on the floor. I think back to *Titanic*. A hanging picture on the wall was his *iceberg, right ahead!* He must have knocked it off while feeling for the light switch.

Oh, my God!

His foot is bleeding. There are bloody early-man footprints everywhere. He is trying to mop up *glass*. I did not know that we owned a *mop*. But, I say nothing.

—*Go, oval superhero, go.*—

I clean up the glass...

I clean up the blood...

I clean and lovingly bandage his foot...

He gets back into bed, curls up on his side and begins snoring, fast asleep. I don't elbow him.

I get back into bed and watch the morning news, which thankfully starts at 4:30 a.m. so people up at that ungodly hour can feel like less of a freak I mean, get a head start on the news.

And I think, on repeat, I cannot believe we are going to be parents... I cannot believe we are going to be parents...

Love,
Mom

GRAPES.

Tuesday, April 13, 2010

Dear Babies,

Today I went to the doctor, *the* doctor, the miracle doctor, to pick up my medical records so I can bring them with me tomorrow when I see our regular OBGYN. (You'll be nine weeks, the size of grapes, time to fire up the 70's time machine, time to see you again!)

Wow, is this thing a tome. I'm talking a file the thickness of Stephen King's *It*. How many times I'd sat in that waiting room fantasizing about this moment. "Good-bye!" blowing air kisses to the office. Giving double peace signs down on one knee. *A sign, to run through, for me?* Instead I got a few hugs, gave a few kisses.—"Congratulations!"—Then the phones were ringing and the nurses had to answer. Women were calling desperate for answers, *I know.*

I turned to the elevator and pressed the button, down.

Inside were more nurses I recognized. I wanted to thank them a thousand times over, above and beyond. Headlocks and noogies were not out of the question. *Come 'ere, ya big lugs!*

They were talking about what to order for lunch. One girl said she had a sandwich of vegetarian turkey salad. *My kind of girl*, I thought, when I could do basic human things like eat food. I debated using that as my opener to join the conversation, but then the elevator stopped at the second floor and they all got off, giggling in a cluster. And I was left standing in their wake as the copper doors closed, eye-to-eye with my blurry self in the reflection. *They're just people*, I realized, *at work, ordering lunch, and yet they do such extraordinary things. . .* I imagined being so happy in this moment, sailor clicking my heels, swinging around lampposts, but instead felt humbled and small. The doors reopened and I stepped into the brassy lobby. I nodded to the sleepy security guard who, despite how many times I'd signed in at his clipboard still showed no recognition. I was anonymous. These people were the world to me, this place and its news my obsession. But I was just one of many passing through. And this is just their job. I swung around the revolving door and there was no parade for me on bustling Broadway. I winced in the bright morning sun. I was tempted to squint up to the second story window. To see if I could meet the eyes of a woman gazing out like I used to while getting daily blood drawn. Maybe I could send her a message of hope, and strength, *you're not alone, keep trying, love, keep trying. . .*

But I walked looking straight ahead only, a forward march into the unknown.

Love,
Mom

Friday, April 16, 2010

Dear Babies,

Your dad and I had to wait an hour-and-a-half at the doctor's office today. He, with his patience of a gadfly, kept nudging me, *"How come every person comes in after us and leaves before us? It's like waiting for you outside of 7-11."* Like the wait was somehow *my* fault. Men, I'd say, except one of you might be a boy.

I started to skim through one of the dozens of baby books that friends, friends of friends, friends of friends of friends, *basically anyone who has had a child and can spell the word friend* have given me. I thought parenthood, like love, was the one thing there could be no book for, and yet there are *so* many of them out there, either written by experts or the opposite of experts—"real moms"—a category which somehow includes Jenny McCarthy.

The Contented Baby.

The Happiest Baby.

Babywise.

To Serve Man. . . no, wait, "It's a cookbook!"

(Sorry, your mom is a *Twilight Zone* geek. Moving on. . .)

I looked around at the other pregnant women sitting uncomfortably in their chairs in our horse shoe of a waiting room. They were reading magazines. Useful magazines with functional titles. *Parents. Parenting.* Informative pamphlets on reserving cord blood. I dropped my head and began reading *Sippy Cups are Not for Chardonnay.* I elbowed your father twice in the ribs and whispered, "glad to see I'm starting with the basics!"

Some people make jokes when they are nervous. It's just what they do.

Love,
Mom

KUMQUATS.

Wednesday, April 21, 2010

Dear Babies,

Last night I was sitting on the couch with your dad watching *American Idol*. Well, I was watching. He had his nose in his iPad the whole time, probably checking email or looking at houses now that we've decided to move to the 'burbs, to not live in a people-to-bedroom ratio of 4:1 and think that converting a closet into a windowless nursery is a *great idea!*

"So the new fun thing of the day is," I prefaced, for everyday there seems to be a new thing happening to this ol' body of mine that I need to warn him about, and fun is open to interpretation. "This is really random, but I looked it up online and it says that it's normal. . ."

No reaction from him.

"I mean, I always had a little peach fuzz or whatever. I mean, I *am* human, and humans *are* animals. . ."

Nothing.

"But, now, it's weird, my stomach is really hairy."

Bingo!

Still nothing.

"Babe?"

Finally, I was rewarded with a side glance.

"Huh? Oh, sorry babe. Bill Blah-blah-blah just friend-ed me on Facebook and I haven't seem him in, like, twenty years." And he dropped his head back to his iPad.

I blinked.

The theme song to *American Idol* resounded through the air.

"Right. You go back to Facebook. That's much more important than your wife turning into Sasquatch before your very eyes."

Happy ten weeks, babies. You are "barely the size of a kumquat." What the heck is kumquat.

Love,
Mom

Thursday, April 22, 2010

Dear Babies,

Today is Earth Day. As a wannabe hippie I was looking forward to it, happy that a formerly nothing "holiday" is now becoming mainstream. When I woke up this morning at 4:00 a.m. I heard it was not going to be a nice day, but by the time the sun rose all those forecasters were wrong. (Note: They often are.) It is *beautiful* out. The Italian ice man is parked in front of the elementary school across the street. I can see him from our kitchen window and on warm sunny days such as this he tortures me so. One day I'm just going to have to go down there and get one. Lemon. Or coconut. No, lemon, since when it comes to ordering food, babies, you should go with your first choice. (That or order what the person at the table next to you is getting. Trust me, you'll always want it.)

I went for a walk in Central Park armed with a bag of stale bread crumbs hidden in my palm. There are signs saying it's against the law to feed the pigeons, but pregnant women are like old ladies like that. We can break the law, wear muumuus and fart in public, *who's going to stop us?*

I was at the far northeast corner of the reservoir, leaning over the railing at the exact spot where I know the turtles like to hang out. They were sunning themselves on a rock when I noticed a family of ducks approaching. The ducks were swimming, dipping under the murky water, splashing and playing. I emptied what was left of my crumbs and watched them eat, lost in thoughts of a house with a yard and being able to go back there and feed the birds with you, like I used to with my Pop. . . until I noticed the ducks were frolicking in a cluster of trash. I leaned over the railing to look closer. Amidst the usual pond scum and algae was an empty jug of milk, a child's yellow plastic toy shovel, the orange cap of a Gatorade bottle.

Suddenly, I felt really sad.

I thought of how everyone talks about "going green" these days, yet clearly people are still throwing trash on the ground. Where do they think that it goes?

I thought about college when I used to smoke and how I used to throw my cigarette butts on the ground. Of all the potentially regrettable things about that time, from bad haircuts to horribly cheesy late-90's outfits to boyfriends (actually, I had none, see "bad haircuts," but whatever), this disgusting habit and thoughtless action is something I truly do regret.

While I try to believe being an adult means not blaming yourself for the mistakes you made when you were a child (*sounds smart, right? Because I didn't say it, but I can't remember who did), as a parent now I feel an extra sense of guilt. You'll be inheriting my world.

It's hard to see beyond tomorrow when you're eighteen. Remember, babies, you gotta think. Footprints get erased in the sand but not in the heart—and definitely *NOT* on Facebook. You want to leave a trail you can be proud of.

Maybe Earth Day functions as a reminder that any day can offer the chance to turn around and make a change, a chance to be a better person. . .

Maybe today is the day I get that lemon ice, too.

Or coconut.

No, lemon. Definitely lemon.

Love,
Mom

Monday, April 26, 2010

Dear Babies,

Friday night I ordered so much Chinese food for myself that the take-out guys gave me four sets of silverware, four little mustard packets, four fortune cookies. Now that I can eat without regurgitating, I eat everything. I sat at the kitchen table devouring my feast—spring rolls, moo shu vegetable, broccoli in brown sauce with shrimp fried rice—reading all the "learn Chinese" words from the back of the fortune scrolls out loud. Maybe you heard them and they've sunk in and you will be born geniuses. Your first words will be spoken in Cantonese.

—Horse carriage: "Ma che!"—

Saturday night, *Ratatouille* was on. An animated movie about animals and food? *Love.*

Sunday I bought $250 worth of granny bras and underwear for myself (I'm a "c" cup, babies, from barely b to a full c!!!) and my first Bella Band. Imagine, a giant piece of elastic that goes around my hips allowing me to wear my pants *unbuttoned* in *public*. I am never going to button my pants again, pregnant or not, at least not on Thanksgiving.

Sunday night your dad returned home safely from a bachelor party in New Orleans with all limbs and his pride intact, and—the clincher!—the movie *Mystic Pizza* was on.

Sometimes when you least expect it things line up and everything goes your way.

Or, maybe the secret is keeping life simple enough so that it just seems that way.

Love,
Mom

Tuesday, April 27, 2010

Dear Babies,

I saw a little dog walking with a stick in his mouth. He looked kind of scrappy, a mutt with some beagle in him and unruly hair. He looked how I feel sometimes, especially when I'm rushing, late for something, in the rain.

Anyway, he was so happy to have this stick. You could tell by the way he was prancing with it, his wet black snout high up in the air, his short stub of a tail pointing out, his soft, floppy ears pinned back.

It's so important to do what makes you happy, babies.

Cut out all the garbage in life and things you do for other people or because you feel you "have to," and figure out what makes *you* happy.

I helped an old man on the street today. He was walking toward me with a cane, bogged down with all of these bags from Fairway, and his shoulder bag was slipping to the ground. I saw a quart of orange juice in there. "Excuse me," he said holding out his arm as I reached for him. I offered to take the bag but he wouldn't let me. I slid it back up onto the lumpy shoulder of his tan windbreaker. I secured him so he that could continue on his way, then watched him walk, folding into the crowd down Broadway till I could see him no more.

He was so cute.

He reminded me of Poppy, whom I miss so much. I miss his tweedy hat. His hands. Sometimes, the mention of a person's name can twist your heart into a feeling, like a towel being wrung.

. . . It made me so happy to help him.

Love,
Mom

FIGS.

Sunday, May 2, 2010

Dear Babies,

You think you have a handle on how many weirdos live in New York City and then you have an open house in your apartment. That's when the true weirdos come out. The super freaks. The mole people crawling out from the rocks they've apparently been living under, or worse, *Brooklyn*.

They come to your apartment and sit on your bed to get a "feel" for the room, bouncing their behinds up and down, up and down. They open up your closets, your refrigerator, and *oh, the humanity*, use your bathroom.

I'll be okay.

I just need to go change the sheets, wipe down everything, dip us in Lysol. . .

Love,
Mom

Monday, May 3, 2010

Dear Babies,

"Really?" your dad asked, breaking the silence of the crowded waiting room of the Columbia Presbyterian ultrasound office. He was in apparent disbelief over how long it was taking me to fill out the doctor's questionnaire. "This is not an essay, babe, *come on.*" He dipped his thick, dark eyebrows over my clipboard, saw the question I was stuck on and exclaimed, "Thirty-one!"

I rolled my eyes at him. My age. Of course I know *that.* "But the question is confusing, *see?*"

—"*Did you use in vitro fertilization? If so, what was the age of the egg donor?*"—

"We did use in vitro," I explained my confusion in not much of a whisper at all. After all, there's nothing to hide. "But we didn't use a donor, we used my eggs. I am the egg donor. The egg donor is me. *Finkle is Einhorn, Einhorn is Finkle.*"

He blinked at me. I blinked back. He could not believe that I just quoted *Ace Ventura: Pet Detective* in a waiting room full of very "adult-like," very serious, very pregnant couples. Everyone was in yoga pants and spongy flip flops. I was in converse high tops and high-waisted jeans. There's a scene in a movie *Dazed and Confused* where a girl in trying to squeeze into a pair of similar pants, pulling the zipper up with pliers. Unbuttoned with a Bella Band, my look as I stood to point out the questionable question, was the opposite of that.

"No one has ever brought this up to us before!" The nice nurse said coming out from her post behind the desk. "Thank you, we'll have to fix that!"

(See, babies. Don't be afraid to open your mouth. Even in quiet waiting rooms where it kind of feels like everyone hates you.)

We were there for something called the Nuchal Translucency Scan. In English, the First Trimester Downs Screening. A combined blood test and ultrasound that would tell us what the "chances" are of you guys having a chromosomal abnormality. *Grrrrrrrreat.* I was tearing up inside even over how to pray for this. I wanted to pray that you are "normal," but then I'd stop myself and think, *is this wrong?* Because no matter what the results of this and every test are, I will love you the same. And—*bombshell*—there is no such thing as *normal.* Nanny says how great that they test for all this stuff now. Back when she was pregnant with me, back in the Stone Age, they didn't even have sonograms, can you imagine? What will they think of by the time it is your turn? From diabetes to genetic disorders, I've been screened for *everything.* (I am a carrier for cystic fibrosis, who knew?) But sometimes I think (kidding, *of course*), especially the night before such a test, *how nice to be having a bloody mary in the living room like Betty Draper right now, oblivious. . .* Because that's the hard part of all this medical stuff that comes with pregnancy, *knowing* how helpless you are. I promise I won't let anything to happen to you, yet I am faced with the reality of test results and circumstances beyond my control. I hate gambling, and it all makes me feel like I'm just rolling the dice. Some babies are healthy. Some are not. And man is it scary. It makes me want to crawl into the corner with my hand on my belly and say, please, God, *not us. . .*

In the end I do put my hand on my belly. I close my eyes. I breath in and out. I do pray to God. I say, *"please, send us strength, and faith."*

I'm beginning to see that as a parent sometimes that's all you can do.

Your dad wanted to cancel this screening—"If we know we're not going to do anything no matter what the results are, then why even take it and get all stressed out for no reason?"—but this test *did* mean an ultrasound, and I wanted to see you. . . and I am so glad that we did.

You guys really look like "babies" now.

It was so amazing to see your two different personalities coming through! (I know, you guys are 1 1/2 inches long, but let me have my fun, okay?)

Baby "a," on the bottom, you're the one who will come out first. You were such a calm little angel. So "chill." You were content in your spot resting your chin on your chest as if you'd just fallen asleep reading a book in the sun. Baby "b," on top, you were nothing short of a maniac, *God love ya*, as my Nan used to say. Non-stop moving and dancing and kicking around—were those tucked forward rolls, like your Auntie Krissy and I used to do in our pool? *Impressive.*

Your father peaked out from behind his phone, recording the whole thing. "They're kind of like two people we know." And I chuckled through my tears, which resulted in this weird kind of snort, thinking of your dad who can fall asleep so easily, hit his spot and be out cold for the night, and then me, on the other hand, tossing and turning, kicking, my mind racing, no rest. . .

You're going to worry about so many things in life, babies, that at the time feel so important. School. *Will I make the team?* I'm so late for this meeting. How many hours do we spend stressing about *work*.

And then you get test results back saying you have two healthy babies growing inside of you, and with this tremendous blessing you also realize you've been gifted perspective. Suddenly it's so clear: nothing else matters in the entire world except for the health of your family. Nothing. That is a big enough weight on its own. Everything else, literally, should get tossed off with a shrug.

Remember, you beg of yourself, *remember to walk the flat-footed steps of a warrior, tossing off the ever-creeping nonsense as I go.*

Love,
Mom

Tuesday May 4, 2010

Dear Babies,

    I got my upper lip waxed this morning and the woman really took a lot of liberties on it. It felt like she was waxing down to my jawline, like I had Daniel Day Lewis' mustache from *There Will Be Blood*. I thought I just had some white fuzzies going on, but apparently not.

Love,
Mom

LIMES.

Wednesday, May 5, 2010

Dear Babies,

"What did you make?" Your father grimaced, entering the living room with his keys still dangling in the front door. So much for, *Hon-eeey, I'm ho-ome!* "It stinks like Benihana in here!"

"Nothing," I batted my eyes coquettishly from my usual post at my desk, slouched down in my chair with my lower back resting on a pillow, my legs wide open, my humpty-dumpty belly sticking up to the sky, practically kissing my laptop. I was lying through my teeth.

Okay, I know I shouldn't cook on the days when we're showing the apartment. For our first broker's open house a few weeks ago I accidentally made a giant tray of baked ziti. To the Italian in me, the apartment smelled delicious. *What person coming through the door at 6:30 p.m. after a long day of work wouldn't love to come home to a fresh tray of ziti?* To the rest of the human race, not so much.—"Babe, it's not apple pie... not everyone's a gavone... not everyone's Italian!"—Outwardly, I had stubbornly disagreed. Inside, I got it, and have since tried to refrain from cooking on nights when the apartment is being shown.

But now that the sight of everything doesn't make me want to vomit ("oh God, spinach!"), all of those food commercials, he doesn't understand! Everything looks so *good*. Totino's pizza rolls. Purdue chicken nuggets. Meatloaf—and I'm a vegetarian! Oh, what I would give for a bowl of Olive Garden minestrone soup! And those strangely tubular breadsticks! My Italian ancestors are rolling over in their graves.

And then I saw that cauliflower commercial... pre-made and frozen in a bag with some buttery cheese sauce... I had to have it.

(Had to.)

I chopped up some raw cauliflower and onions this morning, roasted them in the oven with olive oil, sea salt, a ton of cumin, melted some cheddar cheese and some butter... It was delicious.

"You seriously think it smells like I cooked in here?" I said high-pitched, the cat who not just swallowed the canary but a head of cauliflower with cheese, as I reached for a vanilla scented candle within arms reach...

There are some things your father just doesn't need to know, babies.

{Pause. Blink. Silence.}

But you should always tell me everything, of course.

Happy Cinco de Mayo. How fitting that on this day, twelve weeks, you are now the size of limes.

Love,
Mom

Thursday, May 6, 2010

Dear Babies,

I saw the warning signs coming and yet I chose to ignore them. The huge bags. Losing everything *in* the huge bags, my keys, my wallet. Gum wrappers and old tissues and illegible ancient receipts lining the bottom along with five million crumbs. (What, am I carrying muffins around in here?)

It's official: I have become my mother.

Like her, I've become ridiculously honest when someone asks me a question.

"Ever smoke?" said the white-haired doctor in our living room doing blood work and all sorts of tests for our new, souped-up life insurance we're getting in your honor. He was in a short sleeved button down shirt and a tie, a look you don't see today unless you are a pilot. His white-bushy eyebrows dated him at no less than 197 years old. I wanted to lean in to ask him, "Were you Professor Marvel in the 1939 movie *The Wizard of Oz*?" Instead I answered, "Oh, yes!" too enthusiastically. "In college. Socially. About four, five years, 1997-2001." I was this close to actually taking something to my lips and pretending to light up for him, offering a visual, until I noticed your father maniacally waving his arms and jumping up and down like his pants were on fire in the background mouthing, "NO! NO!" Whoops, I forgot. *You're supposed to lie for these things and make yourself seem as healthy as possible.* I was already wearing an A-line sundress that hung off my body stiff like a lamp shade, if that lamp is the size of North Korea, so that they guy wouldn't know I was pregnant. I got so nervous and abruptly revised my answer.

"Nope. Never smoked."

{Pause.}

He raised his white bushy eyebrows. "Never?"

I smiled the smile of a mean girl who swears she won't tell anyone. *She promises.* "Ever."

With a hard swoop of his pen he checked something on his clipboard. Perhaps "nut job" was a box.

The completion of this metamorphosis into Nanny occurred later that morning when it took me precisely three hours to get out the door.

I went from room to room, starting something, futzing with another something. "Here, I have to straighten up this stack of books for when a broker comes this afternoon. . . oooh, our wedding album!" And there I sat for a good twenty-seven minutes looking at pictures I'd seen thousands of times.

Mother's Day is Sunday and I'm not gonna lie, I've been thinking a lot about what type of mother I am going to be. Don't be alarmed (noting whenever you say, causes alarm) but I never babysat a day in my life. I never ask to hold a baby. Not because I don't want to, but I'm afraid I don't know how. Now in a few months, not only am I going to be handed two of them but told to bring them to my breast to start drinking this milk I'm magically going to produce. *Yeah, okay, because that makes sense.*

But will it though? Will this maternal instinct simply kick in? Will I wake one day like Kafka's metamorphosis and suddenly be a mother? *Do you think comparing motherhood to turning into a cockroach is a bad sign??*

Nanny was twenty-six years old when she had her first baby, Auntie Krissy. I was twenty-six once, I know that's a *kid*. She couldn't have known what she was doing. How did she become the amazing mother she is? How did she always know what to say to us, what to do? *(My God, the teen years, slamming doors, locking myself up in my room blasting Candlebox's "Far Behind," HELP!)*

As a little girl my mom was my hero because I thought she had all the answers. If I could make it to her arms, heck, if I could *hear her voice*, I would feel instantly better. Now she's my hero because I know she didn't have the answers. She was figuring it all out as she went along. I think of this, and it gives me hope.

. . . There she goes again, making everything better.

Love,
Mom

Sunday, May 9, 2010

Dear Babies,

Flowers. Breakfast in bed. Massages. A day of pampering. A day of respect. At least a little butt kissing. These are the images connected with Mother's Day. Not ascending in an elevator a disheveled mess, with hair blown all over in knotty, Medusa-like pieces, a satin babydoll dress caught in unflattering crevices on any lady, especially a newly-showing pregnant one, crooked tights, sore feet, a full bladder, crying alongside a Chinese delivery guy who just let out a loud, ripping fart. . .

No, babies, Mother's Day did not go as imagined.

My day began when I woke up in the spare bedroom of Mimi's apartment in Queens next to your father who upon rising promptly dove back under the gold satin covers and claimed he was about to pass out.

"You're not going to pass out, you're fine."

"I'm dizzy."

"You're fine. You drank too much wine last night."

"I did not, for me I hardly drank any."

I paused in a moment of quiet reflection. He did only have a few glasses and we were both in bed by ten. *He's right, doctor, this much is true.*

"Then you didn't drink enough water. Let me get you some wat—."

{Snoring, as he fell back asleep.}

This was around 8:30 a.m.

I got up, ate a bagel, watched CBS Sunday Morning and read the Post cover to cover (*if you ever want to feel smart, like you can finish a whole newspaper, you can read *The*

New York Post!). "Another 'Real Housewife' publishing a book," I sighed skimming Page Six. As a writer who spends *years* working on projects that might never see the light of day, news of so-called celebrities getting book deals is painful. I eyed another bagel to drown my sorrows, but it was cinnamon raisin. And you either like cinnamon raisin bagels or you don't. *Wah.*

At 10:30 a.m. I went in to check on your father.

He was green. I'm talking Kermit.

His mother wrapped his head in wet towels, took his blood pressure, took his temperature. "The same one from when I was growing up!" he said, as if this were a good thing. A thirty-four-year-old mercury thermometer. I couldn't help but laugh looking at him on top of the decadent maroon and gold satin covers, in his boxers, with a terrycloth makeshift turban.

All tests showed he was fine.

"You're fine," I repeated. "You just need to eat something." Note an Italian's cure for everything: *you need to eat.*

While his mom primped and pomped in getting ready, after all, this *was* Mother's Day, and she had a brunch to make at 1:00 p.m. with your Aunt Shelly in the City, I brought him a big glass of milk (his favorite) and a piece of toast. I took a neat bite of the toast before handing it to him. He saw the missing half-moon but said nothing, proving he must sick.

Upon downing the milk and taking a few nibbles of the toast (to which I thought, *damn, he didn't even notice, I could've had more*), he ran off to the bathroom and puked it all up.

And puked it all up. . .

And puked it all up. . .

And puked it all up. . .

Last night's veal.

"*Ooooph*," we all realized in a Eureka moment, "*It must have been old, that's why they put in on special!*"

(Take note: Be wary of the special.)

At this point I was ready to go in my frilly white baby-doll dress that I had loved in the store but now made me look like a tissue (thanks, Anthropologie!). I had on black tights pulled up to my ribs. High heels. A bright yellow jacket festooned with a few pins, including my Nanny's cameo (my favorite). After all, this *was* Mother's Day, and we were meeting my family for brunch in Pelham also at one. Maga, my Italian grandmother, was coming, and we had been waiting until Mother's day to tell her our good news. I was going to give her this pin that says "Great-grandma of twins" before we sat down to eat.

"I'm sorry, babe, I'm so sorry," your dad looked up from his head in a Waldbaum's shopping bag.

I said it was okay, and I *knew* it was okay, but we were no longer dealing with a rational thinking person here. We were dealing with an entirely different animal: A pregnant woman.

I started to cry, an ugly, snot-snorting cry.

"*I don't know. . . sob. . . where. . . sob. . . I'm going!*"

"*I haven't. . . snort. . . driven a car. . . snort. . . since January!*"

Then, thanks to the amazing schizophrenic powers of pregnancy hormones, the tears magically stopped. I spun my head and turned into She-Devil.

"I'm in *Queens*," I hissed, like Queens was one of the circles of Dante's Inferno.

"I have to go over a *bridge*. I have to go through the *Bronx*. I have to drive home through the City by myself and *park* in our teeny, tiny tight spot in the *ghet-toe* underneath the Boat Basin. I look like a *marshmallow. . ."*

"We can call you a car!" "You can leave your car here!" Your dad and his mom threw options out to appease me, picture tamers tossing steaks into a lion cage.

"What am I, Driving Miss Daisy?" I snapped.

{ROAR!}

In the end I wiped off my tears and fixed my smeared mascara. "I'll be fine," I said poising my chin up high. A third personality entered the room, the martyr. "I'm a big girl, literally," and I slung my bag over my shoulder and marched out the door, singing the chorus to "Freebird."

Let me tell you, it is a very hard to concentrate on being a good driver while using your mirrors and listening to woman shouting directions in an Australian accent at you from your GPS *at the same time.*

Yet Hallelujah, I made to Westchester alive, with only one minor turn-around and pull-over mishap on the side of the road in the Bronx. Maybe one person slammed on their horn and screamed "asshole," but that even wasn't definitely directed toward me.

When I got to the restaurant my family was already there waiting in the lobby. They all looked like they were about to burst. My parents and sister because they were excited, Maga because she was hungry. Right away Auntie Krissy's and Nanny's eyes fell to my growing basketball, further poofing out my dress's already full shape. I realized I had to say something before my grandma did, before she asked me if were getting fat—which she would have no problem doing, kindly pointing out such nuances all my life. (*"What's a matta with your face?"* with acne in the teen years. *"You're awl yellow, you have JAWNDISS!"* after a college night of drinking. Doesn't family sound great?)

"Come on, we're star-vin!" she cried when she saw me.

"Here, wait, before we go sit," I said struggling to keep down the back of my dress that blew up every time someone opened the door. "I have a pin for you to wear. . ." I clumsily pinned the button that was a cartoon picture of two peas in a pod and said *Great-Grandma of Twins* to Maga's black turtleneck sweater.

"Oh, how nice," she said without even glancing down at it, then turned abruptly to head into the dining room, a woman on a mission. One o'clock lunch is really late when you eat dinner at four.

"Wait!" I hollered, startling our hostess. Dishes rattled in the kitchen. A nearby family turned and looked.

Maga finally looked down at the pin, looked up, then tears filled her eyes as her jaw dropped. . .

And she threw her arms around my sister.

"Oh, Krissy! I'm so happy for you!"

"No, Maga, ME!" I quickly spun her around and pulled her into a hug. And we all basked in a moment of nice family awkwardness.

Miraculously, I made it home okay, a remarkable feat considering my GPS took me on every major highway in the tristate area in a matter of fifteen minutes. The Major Deegan. The Hutch. Parkways that sound like cops' nicknames in 80's crime shows. I drove with two hands clenched tightly on the wheel the whole time. My back ramrod straight, no radio on. Instead I talked to you guys. It's the reason people insist on coming to things like big doctor's appointments with you: sometimes it helps to have someone there (even when you swear you're fine alone).

—*"Almost there, guys, we're almost there. . ."*—

Earlier that morning I'd given my overnight bag to your father, but I'd acquired a lot of crap I mean gifts since then. When I finally parked the car I stood above the trunk eyeing my nemesis, a tattered shopping bag full of angular items, picture frames, books, a pair of knee-high boots. At four o'clock, a notoriously hard time to get a taxi in the City (it's when they all change shift), I knew I would have to carry it the ten blocks home. Completely ignoring my instructions to avoid heavy lifting, I heaved it over my shoulder like an old time vagabond with his belongings in a handkerchief on a stick. I took off against the wind, stopping on both the north and south sides of every corner to shift the weight. My tissue dress didn't stand a chance. Around 84th Street I let it completely blow up in a reverse umbrella, abandoning view of my beige spanx which makes me look like a nude Barbie, but totally different.

As with the drive, I talked to you guys the whole time— ". . . *just think of women in the Dark Ages, what they had to go through. . . they didn't even have toothbrushes. . . flushing toilets. . . I can handle this. . . we can handle this. . . "*— breaking thought only once to telepathically threaten the life of a homeless man whose eyes met mine as I passed. "I will beat you with my heel if you touch me and these babies, faster than you can say murder." Meanwhile he was probably thinking, a bag lady dressed like a fairy talking to herself, *such crazies in this town.* (I read an article once about a woman who wore black garbage bags around the City so no one would talk to her, to look crazy to avoid the crazies. This might be something worth exploring.)

When I limped up the steps of our building like a bear shot in the leg, my doorman asked me if I wanted to take up the dry-cleaning.

"Sure, why not?" I said. I am fairly certain Ralph still does not read my sarcasm.

I got into the elevator, heaved a long exhale, and began to cry.

Right before the door closed, a Chinese delivery guy got in next to me. . .

Love,
Mom

Monday, May 10, 2010

Dear Babies,

I had my first encounter with the Pregnancy Police today. I've met a few variations of them already, people I knew, friends of friends bestowing well-intended advice, but this by definition was blatant unsolicited advice from a complete stranger on the street.

"Were you the pregnant woman in class?" A well-kept older woman approached me at the gym as I was trying to bend over to put on my shoes without toppling over like a Weeble.

"Yes!" I beamed, expecting a pat on the back for just doing push-ups and tricep dips, and, like, 10,000* plies (*probably five) like a champ. A congratulations on the babies? A lie about how good I looked? Self-conscious of my unpedicured old-man feet, I quickly slipped them into my boat shoes, but realized, so beat-up and dirty—and *boat* shoes— my cover was actually worse.

"Well, just so you know, you really should be careful. You really should not be twisting."

Pause.

Did she say twisting?

"I'm sorry?" I asked, distracted by a pair of sparkling gold topsiders on the floor. Their owner off, passing the Grey Poupon on a yacht while I, evidently, am the Old Man and the Sea.

"You know, instead of going like this," and she started going "like this," lifting her knees to her elbows and wringing out her waist side-to-side in a throwback to one of Jane Fonda's moves, "you should be going more like this," and her body started doing this uncoordinated motion, kind of flailing about, her knees, elbows and waist all going in opposite directions, if that's even possible. "Or, you know what I mean, open, open, they like to be *open*, babies. Think about when you're squished yourself, you know? And then imagine someone squeezing in on that tighter," during which she recoiled her stomach and started making these inward circular motions with her well-manicured, well-jeweled hands over her groin. "Think. . . *open*," and she spread her inner thighs and her hands apart making sweeping, blossoming motions, an intimate "ah" expression on her face that made me uncomfortable.

Inside my mind raced between *what the heck are you talking about* and oh my God, did I *twist*?

Outside I said, "Yes, thank you. I know."

I know? Did I twist?! I don't think I twisted. There was no twisting. . .

Apparently the woman did not like my answer of "I know," or perhaps she did not buy it through my doe-eyed panicked stare.

"Well, I mean, do you *know* the medical reasoning behind it? Do you understand the science?"

Uuuhh-huh-huh, said my big blue eyes, as if someone had just asked me to draw Washington D.C. on a map. (Seriously, is it Virginia or Maryland, it's just in the middle like that?). She went on as we traveled together down the elevator, out the door, to the corner of Sixth.

"You can't be on your back because there's a blood vessel—"

Whoa, whoa, whoa, who was lying on their back?

"—that runs down your spine and. . ."

Don't let crazy people make you crazy, babies. Some people love to hear themselves talk. They are experts on everything. Don't listen to them. Smile and nod and tune them out. Listen to yourselves. Listen to your hearts.

Meanwhile, I'm sorry if I twisted.

Love,
Mom

Tuesday, May 11, 2010

Dear Babies,

I was always familiar with the book *Great Expectations*, but growing up in the 90's I must admit that I became more familiar with the story when the Gwyneth Paltrow/ Ethan Hawke movie came out based on the classic of the same name. My girlfriends and I, in college we all loved the soundtrack, perhaps as a break from the norm. The late-90's was *not* the best time for music. See a song called "Blue (Da Ba Dee)."

I don't mean to sound negative, babies, but I just want you to know that you have to be realistic when it comes to expectations. Sometimes I have a Pollyanna Syndrome, meaning I can be annoyingly optimistic even when faced with the fact that I am *shit out of luck.* Someone called me a "tool" in an email once and I swore it said "too" with an exclamation point. I'm a dreamer. I shoot for the sky—and I'll never stop! And you shouldn't, either!—but. . . sometimes you expect things to go differently. You expect more from people. You expect them to act a certain way in certain situations. You build up these ideals in your head and then when things don't go the way you imagined they would. . . you feel disappointed, and let down.

I told someone our great news yesterday and I was expecting her to react differently. I expected her to be, I don't know, happier, more excited, for valid sentimental reasons I won't get into now. "That's great," she said flatly in her usual, must-hide-feelings tone, as if I'd just relayed the details of a wacky dream (something no one ever wants to hear about, trust me, even if they seem interested, injecting realistic *oh, wow!'*s). "But nothing with the book, huh?"

"Nothing with the book, huh?" I repeated mockingly later to Nanny over the phone. She knows my writing career is a sore subject these days. Asking me how "the book" I've been working on for the past year is going is like asking a single 38-year-old woman how her love life is at a baby shower. *Just don't do it.* I recently realized the book sucks (whoops!). I can't just go and whip up another one right now. It's a three hundred page fiction manuscript, not a batch of burnt cookies. With wild thoughts of you guys racing through my brain like a drunken streaker all day—*OH MY GOD! WHAT'S GOING ON IN THERE? DOES ANYONE WANT SUBWAY?*—I'm not exactly at my creative best. I'll have to put it aside and work it on once you guys are born. And I will. I'll find the time. Or is that just something I, Pollyanna, tell myself? (See "tool"=too + !)

"Ame," Nanny said with a sigh that says I should know better, "she's not a warm person. *What did you expect?*"

It's not what I expect, I guess it's that I expect.

Today my craving began on 75th Street and Broadway when I passed Fairway and just had to have a red apple.

(Had to.)

By the time I got to Broadway Farms on 84th I was literally foaming at the mouth at the thought of a red delicious. I spent seven minutes picking one out. I was so excited. It was going to be amazing. I placed it on the scale at the register already envisioning my first bite just as the cashier reached down, with her bare hands, to examine its coded sticker.

But before she reached the apple, she had a horrifically gross sneezing attack and hacked up something terrible into her ungloved hands. To top it off, she wiped her nose, both nostrils, with the inside of her palm while snorting. . .

"No, no, my apple, my APPLE! DON'T TOUCH MY APPLE... oh no... She touched my apple..." I broke inside, realizing my bacterial fate.

"Do you want it in a bag or to carry it out?" she asked, cupping my apple in her streptococcus-laden palm.

"Thanks," I said, crestfallen. "I'll take it."

At home I peeled it. Scrubbed it. And then, tossed it.

Instead I ate a peach.

{Sigh.}

What else to do when plans get derailed but mope for a little, then improvise.

Love,
Mom

SHRIMP.

Wednesday, May 12, 2010

Dear Babies,

In retrospect, maybe telling the doctor at our ultrasound that that you looked like alligators was weird.

"Hmm. . . alligators. . . I don't know about that," our doctor said warily.

I bet in the whole history of Columbia Presbyterian, no tear-filled joyous expectant mother has ever gleefully volunteered that her babies looked like gap-toothed seething reptiles. *It's just that you guys were sliding around, swimming with your little arms and legs out to the sides, and your spines looked like the scaled backs of alligators. . .* yeah, you're right, it's still weird. Sorry. I guess there's a first for everything.

There's this scene in *You've Got Mail* where Meg Ryan and Tom Hanks are saccharinely flirting with each other via IM. Their conversation turns to whether they've ever felt like, when talking to someone, they've put out the worst version of themselves. I've felt like that and then some. That I am putting out the craziest version of myself. That so many times after I've opened my mouth I wish that I had not. I wonder, *why did I say that?* I replay the conversation over and over again in my mind.

Here's what I'll tell you guys if you ever feel this way: *You have to say those things, because that's you being you.* And then I can go back and berate myself about it later, *you crazy fool.*

Happy thirteen weeks today. First trimester flies when you're having fun.

Love,
Mom

Friday, May 14, 2010

Dear Babies,

Something happens to your father when he looks at houses. He loses all sense of taste and style and of our likes and dislikes. He sees a yard with some trees in it and a roof joining four walls and goes, "it's great!"

"Babe, it looks like a tree house. . ." I say.

"A meatloaf. . ."

"Henry Hill's house in *Goodfellas*. . ."

With offers coming in on the apartment, we're going to have a lot of these fun open house-filled Sundays ahead of us, if fun means falling in love with a house on-line, then pulling up to it and seeing it looks *nothing* like the picture. It's on a main road. The back yard is a ski slope. No wonder it's affordable, it's next to a power plant, *it's the brain tumor special!*

In any event suburbia, here we come. . .

Love,
Mom

74

Monday, May 17, 2010

Dear Babies,

I've been getting "A.Word.A.Day" emailed to me since sophomore year of college when I had to sign up for the service for an English class.

Fourteen years later, I still love them.

I read each email in its entirety every morning (well, more like afternoon, by the time I sit down at my desk these days). The pronunciations, the brief stories of their etymologies, the used-in-a-sentence examples, the random quotes lining the bottom of each day...

Ockham's Razor.

(That's today's word.)

noun: The maxim that the simplest of explanations is more likely to be correct.

But it was today's quote that struck me:

"Sometimes I wish I were a little kid again; skinned knees are easier to fix than broken hearts."—Anonymous

A broken heart, no, but I do have things worse than a skinned knee I wish I could fix. I wish I could help your father, alleviate his stress and worry about us.

While I am here concentrating on getting enough water (how can I properly hydrate three people when I can't even water a plant) and eating fruit like an animal (literally, ever since I saw those bats on some nature show ferociously devouring mangoes off a tree), he is in full-on provider mode. Trying to get this apartment sold and a house bought for us before you guys arrive this fall. A nice house for us to raise our family in. Maybe with a front porch. Four bedrooms. An eat-in-kitchen. Walking distance to the train. *Can we get a Victorian? Are beach rights too much to ask?*

Our accepted offer on the apartment fell through. So now we're back to square one. *Open houses, realtors, brokers, daily hypothetical mortgage calculations.* I can see the wheels turning in his mind, *"say we only sell the apartment for this and then we're left with that and that means we can buy a house for a max of this. . ."* He says that he's fine but I can hear the stress in his voice.

He wants the best for us, and he feels like he can't get it.

(I know that feeling, too, babies. I know that feeling, too.)

I wish I could just give him a band-aid.

Love,
Mom

LEMONS.

Wednesday, May 19, 2010

Dear Babies,

Oh the utter delight that filled my heart when I walked past this morning.

The hustle and bustle of workers outside. . .

The sheets of brown paper lining the glass windows. . .

The polished light-up sign already in place. . .

I can't believe the good fortune that is smiling down upon us.

Ollie's, babies, my favorite Chinese restaurant, is opening up on our corner!!!

I am going to be there every day!

Already I know exactly what I will order when it opens: broccoli in brown sauce—*not* garlic sauce, you have to specify—brown rice and a spring roll.

I've been thinking a lot about egg rolls lately. I remember loving them as a kid. I used to eat all the delicious shredded insides and never touched the shell. I remember my family would reach over the table when I was finished, pick up the two perfectly hallowed out deep-fried pockets and bring them to their eyes as if they were binoculars, and laugh. "Yup, not a crumb in sight!"

Nobody taught me to do this. I didn't see it on some show. This was a characteristic—okay, quirk—I developed completely on my own. . .

I can't wait to see what surprises you'll have in store for me, babies.

Fourteen weeks today. You guys are the size of lemons. I'd say this calls for Chinese food, if only I weren't so sick from lunch: two hard-boiled eggs dipped in French Dijon mustard, five falafel balls covered in tahini, one-and-a-half extremely sour pickles, and a mango.

Yikes.

Love,
Mom

Thursday, May 20, 2010

Dear Babies,

I admit it, time and space are not my strong points. (I'm always late, and damn those door knobs that seem to jut out from nowhere.)

Perhaps this would've made me a great astronaut, up in space where such nuisances don't matter. I could float about weightlessly, stuck in a pod with Ripley from *Alien* and wake up fifty-seven years later on some planet: "I've been up here how long? Wow! *Time flies when you're flying, huh there, Rip?!*"

But unfortunately, my dear babies, here on Earth I remain challenged.

Your father told me to be ready by one o'clock today when the realtor was coming over with a photographer to take pictures of the apartment. Around 11:45 a.m. I had an intense craving for shrimp. Forget looking up on-line if shrimp were "okay" for me to eat. With the time crunch I'd play Russian roulette with mercury poisoning and go straight to Menupages. (I'm such a rebel like that.)

Do you know how hard it is to find grilled shrimp? Just shrimp, just grilled, lightly seasoned, preferably on a skewer so I can then slide them off and drop them into a salad with croutons, eggs, olives, avocados, ranch and shredded cheddar cheese??

Nowhere seemed to be doing take-out. My most viable option was shaping up to be a shrimp burrito from Harry's Burrito's. Blech.

With the beast hungry and the clock ticking, I made an executive decision: I would have to do it.

I would have to go to Whole Foods, a dangerous destination considering I'm unable to go there without spending at least $30 dollars, even on a stealth mission such as this to buy "one thing."

I had less than an hour to get to the store in Columbus Circle and back, clean the apartment, and eat the shrimp before the realtor arrived so I wouldn't accidentally turn into the Exorcist and spin my head and spit pea soup.

. . . But oh, the sensory overload going on in that store! The strawberries! They smelled so *good!* The carrots still had the long squiggly roots on them and green leafy tops! I imagined myself chomping on them like I were Bugs Bunny!

I coached myself through the produce section as a marathon runner would. *Stay on course, stay on course.*

I searched the hot bar, the cold bar, the deli counters, the prepared foods section. No shrimp. 12:15. Crap. I tried to get myself to want other things. I talked to myself like a tired, desperate parent trying to appease a bratty kid—"look, the olive bar, golden sesame tofu, you like that!" "NO!"—The further I got from shrimp, the more I had to have it. Like Tomas deciding to go back to Prague in *The Unbearable Lightness of Being,* "muss es sein, muss es sein? Es muss sein! Es muss sein!"—*Must it be, must it be? It must be! It must be!*

Shrimp, it must be.

Finally, *hark!* I spied the seafood guy.

"A quarter pound of cooked peel and eat shrimp, please!" Nearly drooling I glanced at my watch. 12:25 p.m. *Might not have time to wait for him to prep more, ooh, but it looks so good.* "Mmm, make that a half!"

I moseyed on over to the check-out counter as if I had all the time in the world. An entire classroom of junior high school children—not from New York, you could just tell—got in line in front of me.

12:35.

Five minutes later, I flew out in a panic, a cold (nope, very warm, hot, actually) sweat.

At five to one, I was Magda on speed from *There's Something About Mary*, frantically wiping down everything in the apartment. I opened up closets and flung in jackets and stray shoes. I peeled off my gym clothes and threw on a sundress so I didn't look like a sweaty egg in spandex. Just as I was about to start preparing my mouth watering feast, the buzzer rang. . .

{Bzzzzz.}

Son of a! One o'clock on the nose? Who does that?

I spent the remainder of the afternoon lurking behind the realtor and photographer, casting longing eyes at the refrigerator containing my beloved shrimp. When they staged the kitchen and set the dinner table, I thought *okay now they're just being mean. . .*

The Dalai Lama was asked on the *Today Show* this morning about how we could find contentment, especially in this age with so many difficulties plaguing the human spirit—from war to the oil spill to the economy. He said, so calmly, *"These problems are man-made. Our own creation. So, logically, we have the ability to overcome [them]."*

So many problems we bring upon ourselves, babies. So much stress. We make life so much harder than it needs to be.

Love,
Mom

Monday, May 24, 2010

Dear Babies,

Today is Monday, the type of day goateed musicians in dimly lit coffee houses sing sad songs about.

My dread of Mondays began in high school. I always loved school. I was a total nerd and genuinely enjoyed spending hours on homework, meticulously writing and rewriting whole loose leaf pages so as to avoid any cross-outs. With every test and paper that came back my heart would thump-thump in anticipation, and I would always be so relieved, genuinely surprised to see my usual: 98. But then when I started doing stupid things at high school parties on weekends (hey, it happens, the CW doesn't have an entire network of shows based on it for no reason) I'd lay awake on Sunday nights with such anxiety about facing gossip the next day.

In college, the dread continued as my nerd-dom was replaced by my love of being Social Chair of Chi Omega sorority—and I took my role of going out at least four nights a week *very* seriously. I still did stupid things at parties—there isn't a flight of stairs between all fifty fraternities at Penn State I haven't fallen down, butt first, head first, on my side sliding-into-home-base in a mini-skirt with no tights (you: we're so proud)—but by then I didn't care. My Sunday night anxiety came from thinking about how I was going to get everything I'd put off for that first 11:00 a.m. class done in time. How I'd have to get to the gym to work off that bag of Wow! Fat Free potato chips consumed Sunday at four a.m. Right on the bag it said this product contains Olestra, which may cause anal leakage. (I know what you're thinking: I was pretty cool in college, *right?*)

Then, the real world. . .

One of the main tasks of my first job as an editorial as-sistant at *More* magazine, assisting the busy, busy editor-in-chief, was answering my boss's telephones. No matter how on-time, or on rare *rare* occasion, early, I was, she was always there before me. Waiting. Calling my name. Ready with a list of that day's tasks. "Aim-mee?" "She lives freakin' ten hours away up there in the boondocks," I would huff, "did she fly here on her broom*? (*She wasn't a bitch, actually—at all. Just intimidating. Smart. Successful. Menopausal.) Oh, how I hated picking up that phone. My scary, high-pitched phone voice. Sometimes the Long Island accent I'd worked so hard to suppress during four years in Pennsylvania would come out hard-core, especially over voicemail. "Amy *cawl-ing* from *Maw* magazine." Once I answered with a mouth full of sandwich and almost choked on my hummus when I heard that unmistakable, "Hi, this is Jamie Lee Curtis," speaking to me on the other end. . .

And now, still, I get that sinking stomach feeling on Sunday nights with my mind racing about everything I have to do the next week, especially if it's dark out and I'm not home. But I've developed a trick for helping me cope:

I think about one aspect of the next day to be excited about. Even if it's a stretch. Buying good cheese while gro-cery shopping. Watching last night's *Family Guy* I DVRed. . .

I know people who always seem to be happy, babies. It's not that stuff never happens to them, I think it's the way they handle the stuff.

Love,
Mom

Tuesday, May 25, 2010

Dear Babies,

I felt like I was in a Meg Ryan movie this morning. I had my iPod on shuffle and Wayne Newton's "I'm Looking Over a Four Leaf Clover" came on. (Yes, I am a proud owner of his *Mr. Las Vegas* album, let's move on.) I walked across Central Park South past the brassy Essex House and the breezy tree-lined park and all the glitzy horse-drawn carriages with a springy pep in my step, chin up, smiling at strangers, imagining myself in a small town saying hello to local business owners in a British accent, *of course.*

'ello, Gov'nuh!

I took the subway uptown and reached the corner of 89th and Broadway, and the next song shuffled to Joan Baez's warbling "Forever Young."

May God's blessing keep you always,
May your wishes always come true,
May you always do for others
And let others do for you.
May you build a ladder to the stars
And climb on every rung,
May you stay forever young.

Oh, my God. . .

By the time I reached the second verse I was a blubbering fool, bawling my eyes out with my shoulders shaking standing next to my fruit stand guy who already thinks I'm a little "off" buying enough peaches from him to fill up a bouncy ball room at Chuck E. Cheese's on a daily basis. For a second in his eyes there it looked as if he might have hugged me.

May you grow up to be righteous,

May you grow up to be true,
May you always know the truth
And see the lights surrounding you.
May you always be courageous,
Stand upright and be strong,
May you stay forever young...

I want so much for you babies. I want not that much at all. I want you to be healthy, and happy. I want to meet you, to hold you, to grab your little fingers and curl them around my pinkies, *that's all I want to do.* I want to tell you that I'm here, that everything is going to be all right, that I got you...

I bought an apple and a peach, and Sheena Easton's "Morning Train" off of *Totally 80's Disc 2* came on.

And I went home.

And I ate the fruit and stared out the window at this ugly fire hydrant, scared as hell.

What if I'm a fool to think that everything will be all right. If something happens to you, I will die.

And now my hands and mouth are covered with juice, and I'm just a big ol' mess.

Love,
Mom

APPLES.

Wednesday, May 26, 2010

Dear Babies,

I think I have amnesia, or at least am like the character "Ten-Second Tom" from *50 First Dates* whose mind wipes a clean slate every ten seconds. I walk into rooms and cannot recall for the life of me what I am doing there. And, I mean, the apartment only has four of them, each with a clear function: the kitchen (food), the bedroom (sleep), the living room (TV), or the bathroom (duh). Everyone said this "baby brain" thing would happen and I secretly scoffed at it, saying, *"please, she was always a ditz anyway. . . "*

Now, here I am, Finding Nemo.

I think I have amnesia, did I tell you that?

Happy fifteen weeks today. You guys are the size of apples, two little apples of my eye.

Love,
Mom

Thursday, May 27, 2010

Dear Babies,

I got this very nice lavender-scented "belly oil" as a gift and decided that this morning, with five minutes left to get dressed and leave the house in order to make a gym-class I'd reluctantly signed up for, was the best time to try it.

I stripped down, took in the patchouli-scented oil that reminded me why I could never fully cross over to my hippie side, and lubed up my protruding torso.

"Perfect, four minutes left," I thought walking from the bathroom to the bedroom buck naked, ignoring the slippery ease at which my inner thighs rubbed past each other.

A side glimpse of myself in the mirror revealed that I was glistening like a glossy honey-baked ham.

Yet even then it *still* didn't occur to me that I had literally just basted my body in oil—slick, slick oil—and now had to get dressed.

Nope.

Of course not.

By then the oil had started to slide off my igloo of a belly and down onto my thighs, soaking into my black lululemon pants as I stepped into each leg with a stretch and a jiggle.

Oh. . . oh no. . . oh this is not good.

I pulled on a white tank-top over my already constricting sports bra I was busting out of Chris Farley style, "fat man in a little coat," and felt the oil start to seep through.

Oh. . . oh man. . .

I looked in the mirror and saw a perfectly round circle of wetness had now stained the tank top, and even more oil seemed to be dripping from my belly button.

Great.

I looked at the clock. *If I am going to make class there is no time to wash this stuff off.* I peeled off the saturated white top and put on a black one, hoping that would better hide a stain, and took off.

. . . I should've taken the fact that the woman next to me on the subway platform ran to the next car as the train pulled up as a warning sign, but no, I walked right on.

And then I understood why.

School children.

Everywhere.

Sitting, jumping, screaming, singing, punching. Eating stinky sandwiches out of crackling plastic shopping bags.

Did I say screaming?

And, the train car had no AC, an unbearable fate for any New Yorker, let alone a hormonal one greased for ignition.

I wedged myself to stand in between a fourth-grader named Raul and a pole, dropped my head to my book on my Kindle—*The Happiest Baby on the Block*—and grabbed on. The steel was grossly warm from a previous rider's hands. The car was as hot as a sauna. Any minute now I expected to cook, my belly to combust like a kernel of popcorn. I felt the oil on my belly start to seep through my shirt.

And then I felt the eyes...

I looked down and met the mesmerized brown eyes of a little boy sitting beneath me, gazing up quietly in bewilderment at my round, sweat-streaked stomach as it seemingly leaked goo. . .

Oh, the questions for his poor parents when he got home. (To them, I am sorry.)

I don't always do smart things, babies. I don't have all the answers—or heck, many at all. But I try. And I learn from my mistakes. And sometimes that's just as good.

I'll tell you one thing, thanks to my acquired knowledge you will never try to "streak" your hair at age 13 with Jolen mustache bleach, or put a marshmallow in the microwave.

You're welcome.

Love,
Mom

Monday, May 31, 2010

Dear Babies,

Today is Memorial Day, a day you will come to associate with BBQs and a three day weekend.

But as your father pointed out heatedly on Thursday night, it has its roots in something more somber. We were getting ready to watch *The Office* and *30 Rock*, "my shows," like my grandma used to say about *Murder, She Wrote* and *Walker, Texas Ranger*, when a commercial for Lowe's came on. He jumped forward from his sprawl on the couch and raised the volume. "LOOK! This is that commercial they got in trouble for and now have to pull. . ." And we watched the seemingly innocuous ad featuring a young couple buying an outdoor grill and talking about how Memorial Day weekend is all about having fun.

"And?" I said, still not seeing the FCC-threatening doom.

"Babe, *'having BBQs and having fun*?' Memorial Day is about remembering the dead. Our fallen soldiers."

While my initial reaction was *okay, Captain Serious*, I felt like a chump. A stupid, ungrateful American. "Oh. . ." I said, and dropped my head down to an unidentifiable food stain on my boobs.

I didn't get to watch my shows.

As if on cue I received a phone call from Auntie Krissy telling me that our uncle had died. Suddenly. Tragically. He was only fifty-five.

My relaxing weekend plans involving cookouts and reading books poolside at Nanny's were replaced by a wake and funeral and all the family drama that comes with it. I ate four donuts and innumerable plates of baked ziti back at my aunt's house while enduring comments like, "DON'T

GAIN TOO MUCH WEIGHT!" every time I took a bite, combined with questions about my not eating meat. I haven't eaten it for fifteen years but still, the Italians cannot *fathom* my survival.—"YOU DON'T EVEN EAT PORK CHOPS?" "Well. . . no, because that's meat." "VEAL?"—

As sad as it was watching my tearful young cousins who had just lost their father, thinking of all of those things that they'll never get to do together—*he'll never get to walk my cousin down the aisle, she'll never get to tell him excitedly that she's having a baby, it's not fair!*—we actually had a lot of laughs remembering all the good times we'd had growing up with my uncle. How funny he was. How he could lighten any situation. How he was always the peacemaker and never took sides in our colorful family. His elaborate stories and tales over the years (sorry, dear uncle, but you never played football for NYU. Besides the truth that you didn't go to college, NYU doesn't have a football team). How big his heart was. How he loved everyone, unconditionally.

So, maybe the people behind the Lowe's ad didn't have it completely wrong. We don't have to cover the mirrors and dress all in black. A day of remembering doesn't necessarily have to be depressing. While it hurts to lose a loved one, it's nice to remember the good things about a person's life. To celebrate them, recall the happy times and memories.

My uncle was the first person to tell me that I was funny. I was in fourth grade. I will never forget it, or him.

Happy Memorial Day.

Love,
Mom

Tuesday, June 1, 2010

Dear Babies,

I feel extra crazy today. Is it normal to feel like my insides are being stretched apart in opposite directions? Okay to be crying this much over Al and Tipper Gore separating?

Each week the gap between me and functioning society grows further apart. It's like as you guys grow out, I slip in. I can't talk to people anymore. I am an emotional nightmare. A farting old woman who can't keep her train of thought. How many times can I stop myself mid-conversation and say, "I'm sorry, am I making any sense?" Because I'm not making any sense. Nothing makes sense anymore.

Being pregnant—*that* doesn't make sense. I am growing two humans and what, people want me to talk about the weather? I don't care about the friggin' *weather*! Oh, it's hot? Oh, it's cold? *Well I am growing two humans!*

A truly annoying thing to say to someone, especially a non-pregnant someone, is "you don't understand." But lately I feel as if the world has been divided in two categories: The universe, and me and you and you. No one understands. I even have a hard time communicating to your dad just how (nervous, emotional, uncomfortable, batty, pick one) I feel.

In May 2008 we started trying to have a baby. We didn't know we had fertility problems. This was back when we thought we would get pregnant like everyone else, by a visit from the stork (!). I had it all planned out, how I was going to tell him our good news. I imagined myself taking the test while he was at work. Being Italian and having everything revolve around food, I was going to set the dinner table with three plates. When he got home and we sat down to eat, I was going to wait for him to notice the extra setting and ask, "Who's coming?" And I would say, "No one, everybody's here. . ."

I imagined it being so hard all day, keeping that secret.

Now I know I can survive things harder than keeping that secret. It is a power I am still growing into. The checkout lady at Fairway huffed and puffed at me this morning when I didn't unload the contents of my basket onto the conveyer belt, a New York City grocery store taboo. Her glower said: Unload the damn bananas. Mine: There's nothing wrong with your hands. Pick up the damn bananas and scan them. Go on. Do it. *And she did.* This is indeed a power.

In college I loved this quote, a line from *The Doors* movie, "She dances in a ring of fire and throws off the challenge with a shrug." I aspired to be such an invincible girl. Today I cling to a more realistic image: Miss Piggy on roller skates heading downhill. Flailing. Frustrated. You know she's going to take some knocks but in the end, she's going to be okay.

Love,
Mom

AVOCADOS.

Wednesday, June 2, 2010

Dear Babies,

I am a female, and I am not dying to go see *Sex and the City 2*.

There, I said it.

I've followed the series for so long to the point that yes, I, too, feel like I know the fabulous foursome personally. Each episode makes me happy, the fantastical clothes, the snappy writing, the love-letter to New York City. I saw the first movie on a fun night out with my girlfriends where we all sat in a row, periodically smiling and leaning in to each other as we laughed.

But now, there's something about this one—is it the giddiness? The overt girliness? The cheap, slapstick humor of Charlotte falling off a camel in the desert? Fifty-five year old Kim Cattrall in gold sequin genie pants?—that, I hate to admit, makes me hesitant to pony up the $12.50 to go sit there and roll my eyes in the dark while feeling like an alien for not genuinely howling along with everyone else in the theater.

Meanwhile, last night a friend of mine from college had a bunch of the girls from my sorority over for dinner. Pasta with homemade marinara sauce. Eggplant parmesan. Cheese plates. Delicious, gooey brownies. Mini-cupcakes from Crumbs. We sat around the table, laughing out loud about "the good ol days." Laughing, and at times, crying, about our lives now. Finally, with my eyes rolling back in my head I cut it short and went home around 11:30 p.m., but really I could've stayed there all night.

The gift of friendship is such a magical thing, babies. It truly is the stuff movies are made of.

Happy sixteen weeks. Avocados. We're movin' on up.

Love,
Mom

Thursday, June 3, 2010

Dear Babies,

Last night I had a dream that you were a boy and a girl.

But in the dream I also got a text message from Jim from *The Office* that said "I love u" (and it came up like that, too, JIM FROM THE OFFICE), so let's not rush out to paint the town pink and blue.

I do feel like there's at least one boy in here, though, and sometimes, I can *see* it. I look at your father sitting across from me at the kitchen table and *see* two little mini-me's next to him on either side. Big blue eyes. Thick curly hair. Blonde, like we both were when we were little until we had "the turn," the cruelty of life being that the only time I was a real blonde it was also okay for me to publicly pee in my pants.

—"*And Mommy,*" all three of them in business-like button down shirts, so serious, hands clasped neatly on the table, "*tomorrow we have to be out the door no later than seven and you can't be late and we have to stop at Home Depot and. . .*"—

I'm hardly a femme fatale, babies, but in my past I've broken a few hearts. I know this because I've been told, *you broke my heart,* which then broke my heart to hear.

I believe in karma, babies.

Oh, the irony of a lifetime of getting teased and tortured by bright-eyed boys.

Love,
Mom

Monday, June 7, 2010

Dear Babies,

In my defense I swore we were dying.

Thursday night I looked down at my left leg and no longer saw a calf but one long club from my knee to my foot. (Google-image search "Fred Flintstone," see his legs for the visual.)

"Babe. . . BABE?!. . . Something's wrong with my leg!" I called to your father who was just about to secure his status as a senior citizen by falling asleep on the couch watching Lou Dobbs.

We went online, which is the best place to go if you want to misdiagnose yourself with a terminal illness, and read that the leg swelling could be from this thing called preeclampsia, high blood pressure during pregnancy. If it wasn't better by the morning I would call our doctor first thing. Your father went to sleep and snored. I laid awake on my back all night staring at the ceiling, dramatically praying like Ricky Bobby in *Talladega Nights*. *Sweet Baby Jesus, please let my leg be all right!*

Our doctor's office opens at 9:00 a.m. At 9:01 I called.

"Only on one side?"

"Yes."

"Your left side?"

"Yes."

"Your lower leg from your calf down?"

{Gulp. Swallow. Brace for impact.} "Yes?" *Crap, what is she going to say?*

"It could be a blood clot."

Crap!

I had heard of these things during pregnancy, and they were usually not good.

But after going through a list of questions and other symptoms with my doctor—she had me measure my legs to compare their circumference—she'd concluded that I *probably* did not have a blood clot. I think she said she was "pretty sure." She told me to rest for the remainder of the day, to soak the leg, maybe wrap it in heat, and call her if anything changed.

Now, when it comes to health, you can't tell someone, let alone a mildly insane pregnant someone, "pretty sure." Like, *I'm pretty sure you are not going to die today. Great, thanks!*

I hung up the phone and hauled my ever-growing behind onto the couch. I stacked my feet up on some pillows and stared at my left leg as someone who looks at a puppy wishing it could talk.

Come on, boy, say something, you can do it, are you okay?

After a good four minutes of intense staring in silence, waiting for my leg to spontaneously combust, I decided that I must do something. So I did what any self-respecting pregnant New Yorker would do: I went to get a pedicure.

"A spa pedicure, please?" I waddled into the salon, anticipating the bubbling hot water soak and wrap and massage being just what the doctor ordered, instantly curing me and my imminent death.

I passed on a magazine and even my Kindle and curled up onto the padded high-backed leather seat dropping my head to my iPhone, prepared to research anything and everything about "blood clots and pregnancy."

Only, suddenly, I could not concentrate.

I felt staring. . .

A room full of eyes was on me. . .

I lifted my head slowly. . .

June, my pedicurist's name tag said, was staring up at me and beaming open mouthed ear-to-ear.

I smiled back at her, not showing any teeth like I did as an awkward kid with a bowl-hair-cut in my dreaded yearbook photos, a look not even a purple backdrop with pink neon lasers could make cool.

I felt glares from my right.

I turned.

There were the manicurists. All nine of them. Staring at me. Smiling.

I turned to my left, and met the bubble-eyed glare of a bald baby boy being bounced on his mother's capri yoga-panted lap two chairs to my left. The mother, too, was staring. Everyone was staring. Like, waiting for this magic moment, "oh, LOOK! The pregnant woman is about to turn and look at the baby!!!"

But, I couldn't...

I could not look...

I was in hell.

Not a hell where you go if you do really bad things, just if you say or think bad things sometimes, like how the baby to my left was not that cute and kind of looked like Sloth from *Goonies*. (Something unfortunate was going on with his ears.)

When the mom smiled at me, I had to do it. I had to smile back.

"Cute!" I said, fake, fake, so unnaturally high-pitched-voice fake.

All of the Asian manicurists and pedicurists started talking, not in English, smiling, nodding, even clapping in approval.

I dropped my head back to my phone to continue reading an article on eHow about how if not caught in time a clot could travel up to my placenta and cut off the blood supply for the babies resulting in stillbirth (NO!!) or travel directly to my lungs and instantly kill me (NO!!!).

June from below stopped massaging my legs and paused.

It was obvious I had to give her, give everyone, more. I had to give them what they wanted. I would have to turn and talk to the glowing young mother.

Effing. . . shoot me. . . if this blood clot doesn't kill me first.

"What's his name?!" I asked forcing a huge smile, expecting to hear Harrison or something from this "Upper West Side" mom.

"Yyyyyyohn," she said.

"I'm sorry?"

"*Yyyyyyyyyohn.*"

"Joan?"

"YYYYYYYYYYYYYYYYYYYYYohn, like John, spelled the same, j-o-h-n, but pronounced Yohn."

I can't, I thought, *I'm sitting here dying and my babies are dying and you're sitting here honestly telling me that your mangled baby's name is John with a silent "J?!!"* For a second I thought I had already died and this was indeed hell.

I sprang up from my chair nearly knocking poor June's white Chiclet teeth out. "I have to go!"

I paid and ran out the door like a freak, waving my arms to flag down a cab. "Columbia Presbyterian, please!"

At the hospital I kept apologizing.

"I'm so *sorry* for being *crazy*," I repeated to the ultra-sound technician, even after she told me that I was okay and swollen from water retention. "I just wanted to hear that everything is all right!"

The technician didn't coddle me. She didn't pat my knee and share a chuckle, *honey, you're not being nuts!* Instead she released a little harumph and said, "honey, don't we all. . ."

Outside I called my mother. My number coming up being the equivalent of the Bat-Signal, she answered in a panic.

"HI! WHAT'S UP?! WHAT'S GOIN' ON?!"

"Ma—" I said, finally getting a word in. "I'm just calling to say hi. Say everything is all right."

There was a pause that followed, a sound of silence I will someday come to recognize as relief.

I never told her about the leg scare, because I didn't have to. I knew she'd heard all she needed to hear.

Love,
Mom

Tuesday, June 8, 2010

Dear Babies,

I just wanted to let you know that I used to have a belly button. It was small, not really cute or anything, just kind of there.

It was an "innie."

Right now it's completely level with the rest of my stomach, and looks like a thumbprint on my taut, pink skin. I expect it to pop out at any second like a thermometer on a cooked brown turkey.

In high school I used to show my belly button a lot, sporting a plethora of midriff baring tank-tops and tight, *tight* baby tees from Contempo Casuals.

(Give me a break, it was the 90's.)

(Actually don't, that's terrible, lay it on me.)

In college I pierced it, likening myself to Alicia Silverstone in the 1993 Aerosmith video for "Crying," when, in reality, I was horrified by all the blood, and later was left with this stupid silver ring I had to wiggle and clean with rubbing alcohol every day in order to avoid a scab and infection. (Now that's attractive! Note today is opposite day.) Worse yet, I made poor Nanny cry when she walked in on me in the dressing room at Mandee's and saw it for the first time.

—*"What are you,"* tearfully, *"white trash?"*—

There's a saying I've heard mothers use sometimes with their troublemaking daughters, a threat that hints at what goes around comes around, *"God remembers. . . "*

If you are girls I am screwed.

Love,
Mom

TURNIPS.

Wednesday, June 9, 2010

Dear Babies,

We got a good report today at our "twenty week" anatomy scan, and I say this in quotes because technically we're only at seventeen. That's one of the many great things about there being two of you, we get extra monitoring, which means we get ultrasounds every four weeks, and toward the end, every two. People who don't know what they're talking about love to tell me that because I'm having twins I'm "high risk." To that I say *my ass is high risk!*, which is not funny, or even makes sense, but that's the mental capacity we're dealing with these days. What happens when Beavis or Butt-Head undergoes hormone injections and then gets pregnant with twins. "Cool!" I am not high risk, but simply carrying two babies at once. I am the ultimate multi-tasker. So, hey, everybody (cue Butt-Head), *shut up.*

Your dad really scared me when you guys first came on the screen and I couldn't see it yet from my horizontal post. "Do they have legs?," he said. All I could think of was Gary Sinise in *Forest Gump* as Lieutenant Dan.

Yes, you have legs.

And arms.

Ears.

Noses.

Lips.

Beating hearts with four chambers.

Brains. Kidneys. Diaphragms. We saw it all. . .

I am so thankful for this rainy Wednesday.

Love,
Mom

Thursday, June 10, 2010

Dear Babies,

Watching Tuesday night's DVR'ed *Glee* at five a.m. this morning was a mistake.

I was just so tired, so delirious, and I still am so tired, purely exhausted to the core. I'd only slept about three hours by that point but yet, as much I wanted to, needed to, I could not rest my mind long enough to fall asleep.

I could not stop thinking about you.

How I cannot wait to meet you.

To hold you.

I'd think I was as excited as I used to get as a little girl the night before a trip to Disney World, which would turn to thoughts of

I'm so excited to take you to Disney World!

To watch The Little Mermaid with you...

To take you to the zoo and to see your faces on Christmas morning when you see all the presents with their red shiny bows beneath the tree...

I can't wait to know what your favorite foods are and to give them to you and see your faces light up at the treat...

—So tired, must sleep, stop thinking about it, you'll never fall asleep!—

I looked up at the ceiling hoping to draw a blank slate, but the striped pattern there cast by the shutters in the silvery moonlight reminded me of the tiny ribs I'd just seen in your ultrasound, and the cycle would start all over again.

—I'm so excited, I can't wait to meet you, I just want to curl your fingers around my pinkies, that's all I want to do... —

Finally, around five, I surrendered and turned on *Glee*, thinking it would provide the distraction I so desperately needed to stop these wheels from spinning and to get some rest.

But of course, it was the season finale, and freakin' Quinn Fabray had to have a baby. When you get engaged suddenly every commercial is about weddings. When you get pregnant—or especially when you are trying to get pregnant—suddenly *everyone* else is, the Upper West Side becomes Babies R Us.

I sat up in bed in the dark crying my eyes out while Jesse St. James from Vocal Adrenalin belted out "Bohemian Rhapsody" as Quinn hee'ed and ho'ed and pushed.

At 6:30 a.m. your dad found me in the kitchen reading the Wall Street Journal blurry eyed and slurping Cheerios. "So, do you want to blast *Glee* and cry hysterically in bed at five in the morning again tomorrow?"

"Nah," I said, "I'm good."

Love,
Mom

Friday, June 11, 2010

Dear Babies,

This morning I spoke to my old roommate who lives in Northern California.

Having known me throughout college and lived with me for two years in a basement apartment in Soho, she's pretty familiar with my often bizarre, heavily condiment-based eating habits. (Mustard sandwich, anyone?) She was dying to know my latest cravings.

"FRUIT," I told her, and I quipped at how I sound like a major "pregorexic" when someone asks me how much ice cream I am eating and I reply, all smiley, *Oh! I'm not eating ice cream! I'm eating veggies and fruit!* "I mean, *couldn't you just punch me in the face?*"

"Yes," she answered honestly, "I could." (This is why you need good friends.)

But I'm talking *pounds* of cherries, peaches, mangoes. Nearly whole watermelons. I could de-vine a bushel of grapes like a cartoon cat slides a whole fish through his mouth and debones it clean. Pineapples? Forget it. I would dive to the deep for a bite at SpongeBob SquarePants' house.

Two at a time cucumbers. . .

Heads of crisp iceburg lettuce. . .

"You're eating like my dad," she interjected, "the gorilla diet."

The gorilla diet. . .

And I pictured a giant gorilla sitting behind the glass at the zoo, gnawing on a stalk of celery, then throwing it down, dissatisfied, and starting to peel an orange with its feet.

Love,
Mom

Monday, June 14, 2010

Dear Babies,

According to dictionary.com, the definition of family is pretty generic: *(n.) A basic social unit consisting of parents and their children, considered as a group, whether dwelling together or not: the traditional family.*

Though I think something more like this would be a better fit:

Family (n.): A group of people you love who drive you crazy.

We have another accepted offer on our apartment and the buyers want to close by September 1st, which means in order to have a house to move in to by then we would have to buy something, like, yesterday. *Yikes.* We're not sure if there's anything we want to bid on right now. "It has to be the *right* house, can't just be a 'we need a house' house!" I remind your dad. I mentioned this to Nanny on the phone and said that we might rent a place if we have to.

With that, Grumpah (your Grandpa's new nickname, isn't it great?) got on the phone. "Why don't you guys just move in here? You can have the two bedrooms upstairs! Mom will be helping you anyway, you can save all that money by not rentin'—"

"Dad—," I said, but this ol' Brooklyn boy was on a roll.

"It would be great! Mom could make din-nuh every night—

"Dad—"

"Ravioli. . ."

"Dad—"

"Meatbawls—"

I thought of Steve Martin selling his daughter on a wedding at The Steak Pit in *Father of the Bride*.

"Dad! Listen, *thank you*, but if we're not in a house, we're going to rent."

"Rent?" They said in unison, both still on the line like Nan and Pop used to do when they'd call me at college from their rotary phone.

"Ma. . . you guys. . . I can't bring my newborn twins home to my parents' house with my husband and have him commuting into the City three hours everyday." The silence was thick on the other end, and silence with us is rare. I stopped myself before saying something more (and you'll see one day, how you can regret saying more). . . Something like, *I have to be on my own for this!* We have to be on our own. This will be our bedlam, babies. Our crazy life. Your Dad and I will deal with the chaos of moving and getting settled and whatever this messy, thrilling life continues to throw our way. I can't bring you guys home to the same purple bedroom where I had sleepovers with my girlfriends playing Girl Talk and making prank calls. Where I hung out with high school boyfriends. Where I hid cigarettes in my pompoms whenever I came home from college. That's too many bizarro things for me, from childbirth (how is this going to work? No seriously, *how* is this going to work??) to standing in the exit of the hospital with you guys in two bucket car seats going, "uuh, what do we do now?" No, they mean well, but I just. . . can't.

"Thank you guys," I said, "but really, we'll be fine. There are houses, apartments, even condos we could rent *on the water*. Really, we'll be fine."

There was a pause. A click. We lost Grumpah.

"Well, awl right," Nanny said, changing the subject, her thick Long Island accent in rare form. "There's a good movie on Hawl-mark tonight, 'Amish Wives,'" and she pronounced Amish with a long "a."

"Ah-mish, Ma, Ah-mish."

I got off the phone and heard my own words resounding through my head. *Really, we'll be fine.*

Any day now I'll believe it.

Love,
Mom

Tuesday, June 15, 2010

Dear Babies,

Moderation never being one of my strong points (I mean, there are two of you), I feel like Alice in Wonderland tinkering with "Eat Me" and "Drink Me," swinging between ginormous and dwarf size. I was feeling good this morning so I went to the gym, but when I got back at 9:30 a.m. I was so utterly exhausted I had to lay down on the couch "for a few minutes." When I woke up it was almost one.

"Great," said my eyes coming into focus on the clock. I felt like I'd betrayed freelancers everywhere, taking naps in the middle of the day, *isn't that what we all do?* If I was going to get up and head to my laptop, face that blinking cursor, something would have to happen.

Since I am so good at self-diagnosing myself (see previous "fatal blood clot" entry) I decided that I must need protein. And iron. *Protein and iron, iron and protein,* I sang in a little jingle as I hoisted myself off the couch. Once standing, I eyed the long journey to the kitchen and sighed, poising one hand on my lower back and taking off shuffling my socked feet along the slippery wood floor. "And miles. . . to go. . . before. . . I sleep. . ." I quoted Robert Frost as I slid like an ice skater.

You should probably know that the kitchen was about two feet away.

. . . Three quarters of a bag of spinach later, along with a can of white beans, a bag of sunflower seeds, a vanilla latte protein shake and a handful of cherries—and that's an Octopus' handful, counting each limb as a hand—I now feel as if I could get down on the floor and do one-armed push-ups like Jack Palance at the Oscars back in 1991. Vacuum the entire apartment building on speed like Magda in *There's Something About Mary.* I may tear open my shirt (well, long cotton maxi dress) like the Hulk any second. Tonight I'll head outside and bench press the moon.

I keep hearing our doctor say during one of our first visits, "Just be normal."

Why is that so hard to do?

Love,
Mom

BELL PEPPERS.

Wednesday, June 16, 2010

Dear Babies,

Today is just one of those days when I feel like everything I do sucks.

I wish that you were here to hug me, or rather I could hug you, because I know that that would make me feel better.

Sometimes you just need someone to tell you that everything is going to be okay, even if it's not.

I promise to always do that for you.

Love,
Mom

Thursday, June 17, 2010

Dear Babies,

"Leah's friend wrote a book that's a New York Times Bestseller, do you want to talk to her? It's about a one-eyed cat."

I dragged my eyes heavily across the pitch black bedroom toward the little green blur on the cable box above the TV. I blinked and it came into focus: 6:10 a.m.

Your dad dressed in his suit with his thick dark hair slicked back and his intense blue eyes glowing, hovered over me. I little more with it and I could've said, "good morning, *Glengarry Glen Ross*." Instead I mumbled, "what?" barely opening my filmy mouth.

"It's about a one-eyed cat."

I didn't respond but shut my eyes while squeezing my c-shaped Snoogle body pillow tighter between my knees. I couldn't face the day and my fizzling writing career just yet.

"What's wrong?"

"What? Nothing." *Just that minutes earlier I had been sleeping, for once, and dreaming about deli ham, vegetarian porn.*

"Are you comfortable?"

Oh yeah, my skin is only taut from being pulled in opposite directions. I'm eighteen weeks pregnant carrying around two large bell peppers and I feel like a number 10 whose "1" just swallowed the "0." I'm perfectly comfortable, thanks for asking.

"Yes, babe. I'm fine. Go, I'm fine. Love you."

I heard the door close and then, silence.

I hugged my Snoogle pillow in closer.

Sometimes, it's easier just to lie.

Love,
Mom

Friday, June 18, 2010

Dear Babies,

Today I went shopping downtown.

Normally I would've gone to one of my vintage haunts on East 9th Street, but no, this was a special trip: This was a quest to buy a maternity bathing suit at Old Navy.

There are all the times in your life when you groan *I have nothing to wear,* and then you get pregnant and the seasons change and you can't just open up your box from last year because oh yeah, you could button pants then, and then you actually, literally, have *nothing* to wear.

Last week I tried on my bathing suits for your father to see what I could still get away with. I tried on a zebra print bandeau top and black briefs I had worn in Mexico six months ago. I could barely clasp the top. Maybe Britney Spears in her cut-offs/rest stop phase would say my boobs and armpit fat spilling over were okay, but not I. And certainly not your father. When I turned to the side and he saw my exposed belly he didn't laugh, which I actually would've preferred. He stared in horror. A look of sheer disbelief. *"Oh, my God. . ."* My button-fly denim shorts I thought were so "huge" and would "definitely" still fit? I couldn't even get them up over my knees. I thought it was just my stomach that was growing. Apparently not.

So I sucked it up and went maternity shopping.

And let me tell you, babies, I got the best bathing suit in the *world.* It has giant cups sewn into the boobs that look like two halves of cantaloupes. It pulls right up with ease. It's almost like a dress. Like something the girls on *Jersey*

Shore would wear to Karma. I am Snooki, or maybe I shoved her up my dress. I also bought pull-on elastic waist denim shorts (genius!), stretchy sports bras, yoga pants that sit so low on the crotch they're borderline inappropriate, but aren't thanks to the longest tank tops you have ever seen. Best yet, I bought huge cotton underwear that comes in a pack of six. It is safe to say I am *never* going to wear a thong again.Viva la granny panty.

When "the hunger" set in (and I mean "the hunger," the monstrous growling that hits every two and a half hours like clockwork if I don't have something to eat; I imagine you guys in there with stop watches like Jack Bauer in *24* constantly counting down until the next chow down: "MA! WE'RE STARVING!!!") I called your father to see if he wanted to meet me at Dean's for pizza. And when I say "to see if he wanted to," I mean to let him know that a feast was about to go down in the very near future and he could either bear witness to it or not.

One cold antipasto platter for two. . .

Herb crusted sole. . .

A large square pie half with roasted peppers, half broccoli and olives. . .

Your father had one slice of pizza.

I ate the rest.

The only thing left were the lemon slices on the fish plate and the prosciutto on the platter.

On the way home we stopped at Godiva where I bought what looked like an ice cream cone filled with six beautiful, plump, chocolate covered strawberries. I'm eating them now as we speak (er, write), chasing each bite with a gulp of cold milk. . .

You are being born into a world where badass rappers can name themselves after squares of frozen water and become actors (see "Ice Cube") and as that great man once said, with assertion, "Today was a good day."

Love,
Mom

Monday, June 21, 2010

Dear Babies,

I just want you to know in case you are super-geniuses and can hear and comprehend everything I'm thinking, that I really am a calm, tolerant person.

Really.

Stop snickering.

I swear.

Those things I thought earlier today. . .

Watch it, fat boy, there's room for only one wide-load on this train and this seat is mine! (Quietly fuming to the chubby 12-year-old boy on the downtown 1 this morning.)

Really, hooched up European girl probably dually breaking child labor and immigration laws with your micro-mini denim skirt and gladiator sandals coiled up to your vagina peddling bicycles? Do you really think I want to rent your bike? Are your fringe bangs in your eyes, can you not see? Do I look like a tourist who happened to consume Sixth Avenue in the stretch between 57th and 58th streets? (To the bike peddler on 59th.)

Call number 10, call number 10! (At Maoz, my favorite fill-your-own falafel pita place).

—"NUMBER 11!"—

What the??? Did they skip me? I waited, waited, waited, eyeing the fixins bar, planning my course of action: Pickles, beets, tomatoes and cucumbers, red cabbage, cole slaw, tahini, and yogurt sauce.

—"NUMBER 12!"—

Son of a! Are you kidding me? They must have skipped me. "Excuse me?" I waddled up to the cashier and handed over my ticket. "Hummus and hardboiled egg?"

The stern looking woman grunted without looking at my order. She didn't even check with the kitchen. "It coming," she prophesied.

I went back to leaning against my garbage can, waited, waited.

—"NUMBER 13!"—

COME ON! I'M FREAKIN' STARVIN' OVER HERE! I'M ABOUT TO FALL OVER! I'M SWEATING IN PARTS OF MY BODY THAT DON'T EVEN HAVE SWEAT GLANDS! FALAFEL NAZI OVER THERE DIDN'T EVEN CHECK! IT NO COMING!!!

"I'm sorry, I just want to make sure—" I said sweetly, sweetly, ever so super sweetly. This time a surly man in a flimsy paper hat looked up over the partition from the kitchen. I smiled. He flared his nostrils—*maybe he has an itch?*—and angrily slid my pita through.

"Number. . . 10," the prophetic cashier mumbled hastily, handing my pita pocket over as if it pained her. In my mind she now has a mole.

"THANK YOU!" I beamed, trying to be so over-the-top polite, feeling guilty for what? She lifted her eyes above my head and beamed to the next customer, happily taking her order, "Hi! Welcome to Maoz!"

What did I do? I thought as I clutched my pita with two hands like a choir boy holding a candle. I kept my head down while loading up on pickles. . .

Deciding I needed something "fun" to wash that down, I went to buy a smoothie from the deli across the street. I asked the woman behind the register what type of berries were in the Wild Berry Blast.

"Ummmmmm," she huffed with a sigh, rolling her eyes, chewing her pink blob of gum with her mouth wide open. I watched it rotate around and around like a lone sock in the window of a washing machine. "It's got. . . berries. . . like, strawberries. . . raspberries, I think."

I thought: *Listen, clone of Tami from* The Real World, Los Angeles, *or is that dating myself and should I say who is now on* Basketball Wives, *why don't you know this? This is your job. Your job is to ring people up, and to know what's in the smoothies. It's not like I asked you what to do about the BP oil crisis. Don't take the fact that you're miserable at your job out on me; we've all done our time with things we don't want to do. Be human. Be kind. Be the best smoothie maker you can be. If you don't know the mysterious contents of the Wild Berry Blast, make something up. I mean look at me, I'm going to order one anyway!*

I said: "Okay, that sounds great, thanks!"

. . . So, I'm sorry, babies.

Maybe it's the heat.

Maybe the world is full of idiots.

Maybe I'm the idiot in the center of it all.

Damn, I wish you could talk.

Love,
Mom

Tuesday, June 22, 2010

Dear Babies,

I think I need some corn-on-the-cob.

I'm a nervous wreck about our doctor's appointment tomorrow. The usual. Hope you're still here. Hope everything's okay. Hope I didn't unknowingly do something stupid to screw this up. I totally get why Tom Cruise bought Katie Holmes that ultrasound machine. I would fire up that bad boy in my living room right now, watch *Jersey Shore* all lubed up with goo. I keep telling myself it won't be so bad once I start feeling you kicking. But that's what I always say. *Once I'm twelve weeks, once I do this test, once I reach the next trimester.* There's always going to be one more thing to worry about, isn't there? My poor mother, how on earth did she survive the college years.

I'm so nervous about this house inspection tomorrow. Yes, babies, we bought a house. Not like a bag or a shoe, but a *house*, a pretty big thing to have buyer's remorse on. I hope everything goes okay.

Heck, because of our doctor's appointment I can't even be there for it. I really wish I could to at least see it again. I can't remember, what are the closets like? What was the floor in the living room? Will my desk be able to fit by that window? Is this normal, that you bid on a *house* and then you don't see it again until you move in? Your dad and his mom and uncle are all going. I know it's silly, but I feel very left out. Like they're saying, *it doesn't matter if you go or not since you don't know anything about house stuff anyway.* Okay I don't, but still. *I* should be the one going (and tuning out the inspector while daydreaming about paint colors and lampshades). Maybe I'm just being witchy because on top of the stress of having a baby (*two), I'm moving out of my beloved New York City into the *'burbs*. I'm buying a *house*. What am I going to do with a house? Can I take care of two babies and a *house*? Husbands in the 1950s used to carry their new brides over the thresholds of their new homes, I think for luck. If your father tried to lift me right now, he would get a hernia. I hope you're not supposed to do this for luck.

A teenage boy came up to me while I was examining eggs in the grocery store this morning. He asked me for money. Was he starving while I agonized over which type of eggs to buy for you guys? *Brown? Organic? Cage-free?* I envisioned the lone twenty dollar bill I had in my wallet, but I couldn't just hand that over to him, *right?* What if he was going to buy drugs or something? I told him I didn't have any cash on me... Still, *what if he really did need something to eat?* I hate how living in the City has made me hard.

Maybe in the suburbs moral dilemmas don't happen at the grocery store.

Maybe that'll be worse, with my plush green lawn and pizza night on Fridays, out of sight, out of mind.

That's why, after a day like today, heavy on the mind, I really think I need some corn-on-the-cob right about now. Crisp. Juicy when you bite into it. Golden yellow with butter and salt.

It reminds me of summer, of being a kid, when people just told me what to do and I listened.

Love,
Mom

HEIRLOOM TOMATOES.

Thursday, June 24, 2010

Dear Babies,

Don't be overwhelmed, I know we talked about a lot of stuff at my "mom meeting" today. Strollers. Bouncer seats. To bumper or not to bumper. I don't know what half this stuff is, babies. And I don't mean "what brand should I get?" I mean like if a television set just fell from the sky and landed in front of a Bushmen—I literally have no idea what this stuff is. A swaddle. An ExerSaucer. A Boppy. These words are not part of the English language yet every mother seems to toss them around freely. *Congratulations, you're pregnant! Now learn our code language, "Momese," and acquire a set of secret skills rivaling that of an assassin.* Swaddle is both a noun and a verb. Oh man, I need flashcards.

I sat at my friend's apartment today with a pen and pad in hand frantically taking notes as she spoke. *"You're going to want this because. . . you don't want to do that because. . ."* All the while nodding my head and saying *okay.*

Finally when she rose to change her baby's diaper, and I watched her move her hands so swiftly around that changing table and all the products and that diaper genie thing, I raised my hand and asked, "How the *heck* do you know how to do this?"

She laughed. "You'll figure it out!" And there was something about the way she laughed that reminded me of a man jumping out of an airplane to cure his fear of heights. "Don't look down!" says the instructor to the panicked diver, slapping his parachute-backpack before pushing him out the door. . .

After one and a half paninis I left with heartburn and a monster case of incompetence. I hard worn this billowy navy tank top from Anthropologie with a white neckerchief tied around the collar that I'd thought was "cute" and now made me feel stupid. Like a fat, stupid, inadequate-as-a-mother person in Popeye's shirt. As I walked uptown toward the 1 train, burping up spicy black bean dip, I decided I wasn't ready to go home yet and then I saw it: Century 21. What better remedy for self-pity than shopping. Before I knew it I was trying on sunglasses that made me look like a cartoon owl. Getting a hold of myself, I left without buying anything but did use the air conditioned bathroom on the way out, so the trip was not a total loss.

Back outside I crossed the street and then I saw it. The other it: The World Trade Center. A site currently known as Ground Zero that you will come to know as the Freedom Tower, that I will forever know as the Twin Towers. I paused and crouched a little to peak through a chain link fence. I watched the construction. One of those big yellow trucks was hard at work lifting mounds of dirt, causing so much dust I coughed and had to look away.

I pressed my hands to my belly and continued toward the subway, aware of the noise of the trucks and the banging growing fainter as I walked.

Somehow I guess we do all figure it out, for life does go on and on and on.

Love,
Mom

Friday, June 25, 2010

Dear Babies,

I used to write movie reviews for *Seventeen* magazine, did I tell you that? When it comes to movies, I know what I'm talking about. Highbrow film? The arts? Cinema? Heck no! I mean me, head-to-head against a frat boy quoting Will Ferrell lines or eighties movie trivia, I will win every time. My specialty is Bill Murray. (Aw, it's okay, you can be proud.)

I had a very Ripley vs. the alien moment from *Aliens* today. Before you say, *what?*, I'll explain.

I was in the bathroom when I felt the presence of eyes upon me.

God?

No, it was a mosquito. The biggest mosquito I have ever seen with spindly legs at least three inches long and a wingspan of the same. It was crawling along the floor from my feet toward the hairs behind the sink. (Hey, sorry, I would clean if I could bend over.) This bad boy has definitely been sucking blood since the Stone Age. He definitely has some T-Rex in him. I contemplated keeping him and mating him with a frog and starting my own Jurassic Park.

But no.

Poised to be squashed by a white clump of toilet paper, this thing held eye contact with me and looked right into my soul, *I swear.* I blinked at it. I leaned in closer. It didn't move. It was then when I realized, *this he is a* she. *This thing is somebody's mother, this thing has a mother.* Like Ripley and the Queen alien in the movie, *we were two mothers facing off.* However unlike the movie, my life was not at stake, nor was the sake of mankind. Having some liberties there, I decided that I must save it.

I hurried to the kitchen and drew back the shudders. I opened the window to prepare for the moment I would toss the mother-saurus back into the world, albeit from four stories high where she would probably plummet to her death, or fly right back into the apartment through the open living room, but whatever, *I would try*.

I grabbed two plastic cups from the pantry.

I scooped it up and trapped it in, ran back to the window and stuck out my hands and *whoosh*, set it free. . .

Perhaps because of this very movie moment, I suggested to your father tonight we go see *Cyrus* starring John C. Reilly and Jonah Hill. "The movies?" he said, like I was suggesting we go out on a bright summer Friday evening to the Holocaust museum. "It's gorgeous out!"

He does not seem to understand that sun+heat does not = gorgeous to me. It means my back hurting and my feet swelling and my legs feeling like they're melting into the pavement as I walk. It means an attractive band of sweat forming between my belly and my boobs that doesn't trickle down, but instead accumulates there, like a stagnant pond.

All I want to do is sit in the air-conditioning and eat popcorn.

Technically the first movie I ever saw in a theater was *Airplane!* My parents sat me on their lap when I was six months old. ("That explains a lot," your dad says, and when I show you the movie one day with lines like "Surely you can't be serious; I am serious, and don't call me Shirley," you'll see why.) When I was two Nan and Poppy took me to see *The Great Muppet Caper*. I can honestly say I remember that day, maybe not the specifics, but the feeling of safety and warmth. Perhaps for this reason I've always loved the Muppets. I've felt a special kinship toward Kermit the Frog.

(When it comes to Muppet characters, everyone thinks they are Kermit, but *I* really am. Don't let your dad try to tell you I'm Animal, either.)

Jason Segel has written a new Muppet movie set to release next November. You'll be a little over one year old. In our very own Hollywood ending, I'll be getting us tickets for three.

Love,
Mom

Monday, June 28, 2010

Dear Babies,

It is hot. . .

Hooooooooottt. . .

I'm pretty sure my torso is now one giant hard-boiled egg.

I made it to the gym today. Made it through class. Made it out the door after to the corner of 57th and 6th where I had to take a little breather against some scaffolding in the shade.

Then I made it one block farther to 6th and 58th. . . stopped. . .

Sixth and Central Park South. . . stopped. . . hunched over, clutching my back, panting like the furry golden retriever on a leash at my feet.

"I hear ya, buddy," I said meeting his sad, black eyes.

I looked up at the towering Columbus Circle buildings in the horizon, the subway there my destination. It looked so *far,* like a castle in the distance. *Where was the flying purple dragon from* The Never Ending Story *to come save me? Atrayu?* If there's ever a time for it to be easy to leave New York City, it's summer. The streets stink like garbage. The stench of fresh hot horse crap wafts from the carriages lining Central Park.

Step, step, step. . .

I made it under scaffolding hanging over the Essex House and heaved down onto a rusty, rickety bar holding it up.

"No, no. . . you sit here. . . better. . . better," a nice uniformed doorman hosing down the pavement suggested, pointing to the ledge of a nearby potted plant. I wondered if I asked him to squirt me, would he do it.

"No. . . thanks. . . I'm okay." At the rate I was going I was never going to make it home. I peeled myself up off the bar and pressed on, taking in the last few seconds of ice-cold air blasting out in bursts from the brassy revolving doors, along with jazzy big band music playing "Stormy Weather" from the lobby, which is funny because that was my Nan's nickname for me. (Especially in the morning when I can be grumpy. Note: Don't talk to me before coffee.)

It wasn't until I finally made it to the subway that I decided to flag down a taxi. One look into the black hole of the mouth leading down to the station and the thought of shuffling into the swampy air there was too much. I hid my torso behind a parked car and raised my hand up, having been warned taxi drivers, those gems, don't like to stop for very pregnant women. (What, they don't want water breaking in their car? When I know for a fact vomiting 22-year-old's falling out of Dorrian's are fine.)

Once inside a car I slumped down into the backseat—*hallelujah, the air conditioning works!*—and I turned my head toward the trees as he drove up Central Park West. In the quiet I remembered, *you might be able to hear things now.* So I took out my headphones and placed them on my belly. I flipped to the next song on my iPhone, a crap shoot since it was on shuffle and my collection is eclectic, at best.

Accept's "Balls to the Wall" came on.

But strangely, while it wasn't the soothing Van Morrison "Into the Mystic" I had hoped for, it felt right in the moment.

I kept it on.

Love,
Mom

Tuesday, June 29, 2010

Dear Babies,
You know they're made in Taiwan, right?
And along with the reeking judgment came a severe eyebrow dip.

I merely mentioned to a friend in passing that I was going to order your cribs from Pottery Barn, and now here I am, lost in a minefield of Google, looking for Amish cribs and hand-made wood furniture online. (There are quite a few retailers, AmishOak.com, AmishEtc.com, AmishOakInTexas...)

No, I didn't *know*. I mean, yes, I know the good people of Pottery Barn aren't whittling wood in a barn back there, but no, I did not stop to think where their furniture actually comes from. Or if it were even possible for a crib to be "bad," unless, of course, its hand-carved by Jebediah. I DIDN'T READ THE OUT-DATED CONSUMER REPORTS BOOKS YOU AND SEVEN HUNDRED OVER PEOPLE HAVE GIVEN ME, OKAY? IS THAT WHAT YOU WANT TO HEAR?!

I need to stop. I need to tune everybody out. I need to remember that I grew up in the 80s, a decade that probably single-handedly destroyed this little thing called the ozone layer. I survived Styrofoam, second-hand smoke and lead paint on my toys. Helmets, *for bike riding?* Try a seatbelt in a car would've been nice! Do you think the Easy Cheese I used to spray into my mouth from the can was organic? My butt.

(No, I mean after years of spraying that Easy Cheese into my mouth, you should see the cellulite on my behind.)

I hate everyone, which really means, I hate how everything I do now brings up my fear of failure as a mom. There is so much pressure to "do the best thing for your baby." So many opinions. So many right ways. I feel like I can't even buy a crib without potentially making a catastrophic mistake and receiving judgment. *Of course* I want what's best for you guys. I have a coupon for Pottery Barn, and I think the Kendall crib is cute, *is that not enough?*

I'm frustrated, and this stupid segment on the Today Show is caught in the crossfire. Jenna Bush Hager is a heartbeat away from getting a banana peel chucked at her head.

Twenty weeks tomorrow. Mid-way. We've come so far, but it still feels like there's a long way to go.

Love,
Mom

BANANAS.

Wednesday, June 30, 2010

Dear Babies,

Nanny and Auntie Krissy keep texting me pictures of shower invitations.

I'm not gonna lie, showers are not my thing.

When they first brought up the event, a few days after we found out I was pregnant, mind you (showers are their thing), my shoulders went up and I immediately started in on my list of "no's."

It will not be a surprise.

There will be no games.

There will be no diaper cake.

No balloons.

No little white candy coated almonds given as favors in bags of tulle.

I will not walk into a room of baby pink and baby blue. . .

And then, it hit me. . .

"You guys," I told them, abruptly changing my tune, "if I get to the point where I'm lucky enough to be having a shower for two healthy babies, then go for it. Go nuts. Let's have a rager. Wrap me in tulle. I'll spew almonds like a fountain. *Do you whatever you want to do.*"

This one invite they just sent me is really weird. There's an old school stroller on it that looks like the creepy one from *Rosemary's Baby*, and yet, with all of my heart, I say thank you.

Love,
Mom

Thursday, July 1, 2010

Dear Babies,

This weekend is the Fourth of the July, my third favorite holiday after Thanksgiving and Christmas. (Groundhog Day comes in at a close number four. We have a national holiday, babies, based on a fictional weather-forecasting groundhog named Phil. We're one of the most civilized societies in the world and we note this on our calendars. Just thought you should know.)

My first front page story ever was on the Fourth of July.

It was in "The Daily Collegian," Penn State's daily newspaper, in 1999.

"There's something about the Fourth of July that brings to mind a good time," it began, and man was it terrible.

But I was so proud, seeing that byline. I didn't care that it ran due to slim pickings for news at the time: dead summer in Centre County, PA. That my editor was probably choosing between my story or something from the police log the night before. "Summer session student pees on fire hydrant and steals plant." I think there was a whole paragraph in my article about hot dogs. One of my sources was a six-year-old girl.

I sent home about thirty copies of that paper. Folded. Stuffed into a big manila envelope. Taken to the post office and mailed. When Poppy died, we were cleaning out his house and there in a bedside drawer were about ten of them, still so neatly folded though yellowed and old.

You would've thought I'd won a Pulitzer prize.

See that everybody has a stories, babies.

I don't mean go and write about it like I do. I mean see this with your eyes. See that as different as we all are, we all have inner battles. We all have heartache. We all have dreams.

For this reason, treat everybody kindly.

Do this and you'll always make me proud. As if you'd won a Pulitzer. As if you wrote a cheesy article about the Fourth of July.

Love,
Mom

Tuesday, July 6, 2010

Dear Babies,

Your father put me on house arrest today.

"Babe, it's 101 degrees out, please, do NOT go outside, okay?"

"I know," I said high-pitched, which when said in that tone blatantly means *I'm lying!* I was already visualizing my walk around the reservoir in the park. I haven't seen the turtles in so long.

"I MEAN IT!" he scolded, as if he could see my bubble thoughts. "Babe, *please*, just for today, it's so hot out, stay inside with the A/C on."

Upon further thought this really was not a terrible request. I crossed off the walk from my internal checklist, but, like the classic Bugs Bunny episode where a hungry Bugs is stranded on a deserted island with a fat guy and a skinny guy and sees them as a hamburger and a hotdog, I eyed your father's rolled up newspaper in his hand and thought, pita sandwich, *hey that looks good.*

"I need to go grocery shopping!" I called after him, proactively confessing to my jailbreak.

"That's fine—but go soon, before it gets too hot—and get the bags delivered!"

"Okay."

"Promise?"

"Yup."

Note how I never said "I promise." I may be Humpty Dumpty dangerously close to a griddle but I still cannot justify the convenience of having some guy carry home my groceries when we live right around the corner. Maybe at seven months I'll start accepting the fact that I can't physically do the things I used to, schlepping included.

(Nah.)

With unshaven armpits I threw on a long yellow tank top, a banana in shape and color, over a pink sports bra and purple cut offs I'd made from sweatpants. No make-up. *I'll be in and out, who's going to stop and look at me?* As I headed out the door I plugged my earphones in and slid my silver-lensed Ray Ban aviators on, secure in my thick, brown spongy flip-flops. It was the type of look I imagine stars love getting caught in so they can prove to the world they *are* just like us, they can look like crap, too.

At Barzini's I loaded up on fresh fruit and vegetables, pre-made salads and chicken for your dad since he also forbade me to turn on the oven, another not so bad request: "Don't cook!"

"I'm okay, I got it," I protested to the cashier as I struggled to hoist the jam-packed black cotton bag I use for groceries over my shoulder. Forget nice little reusable shoppers from Whole Foods. This bad boy is a huge shoulder bag from Urban Outfitters emblazoned with a giant wolf's face on one side in soft, mystical colors, purples and silvers and cornflower blues, and I wield it like a biker named Moon Shine. Only once I exited the store I realized, *I don't got it.*

Not only was the heavy bag cutting off the circulation in my arm—*what the hell is that, the potatoes?*—but I'd forgotten to buy everything I'd gone out for in the first place.

Three layer bean dip, check!

Eggs, milk, OJ... crap.

I hobbled into a Food Emporium a few doors down. "Sweet Lord Hay-Zeus!" I said aloud, spying a shopping cart I could dump the bag in and push.

Eggs.

Milk.

OJ.

Ooh, Life cereal...

Ooh, the frozen aisle...

I'm like a dog walking down the street when I'm in a grocery store, distracted and tempted by everything. My eyes lit up with delight at the sight of waffles, soy chicken nuggets, pot pies, ice cream.

I hooked a sharp right with the cart to head up the next aisle, and crashed it directly into a giant, multi-tiered display of red-white-and-blue chocolate covered pretzels. The whole thing came tumbling down.

A million little pretzels.

Plastic containers.

Metallic red-white-and blue flags.

Streamers.

Cardboard shelves.

If Jaws attacked Aisle Thirteens the way he did lagoons, this damage still would've been worse.

"Oh... oh God... I'm so sorry!" I cried.

The entire store came to a standstill. Customers. Butchers. Deli slicers. Stock boys. An old man reading the back of a box of cheese blintzes. Even the music, the awful soft pop I normally loathe yet find myself singing along to while I squeeze melons (Jessica Simpson's "With You!") seemed to freeze.

All eyes were on me.

"I'm so sorry!" I cried again, both hands still tightly clenched on the wagon, my knuckles and face white as I stood amidst the wreckage.

"It's okay, honey," a female butcher came hurling out from behind her counter in her dirty whites. "It wasn't you, girl, it's the baby!" She laughed as she bent over, picking up a pinkish-red pretzel off the mound and popping it whole into her mouth.

"It's TWINS!" I offered, as if the fact that there were two of you would make it any better.

"It's EARL's fault," I heard a disgruntled man's voice grumble to my left. "Damn Earl and his decorations. I always tell him, why he gettin' all fancy for? Look at these corners, here, here," as the angry elder pointed to a tower of Coconut Water, to a pyramid of Stove Top stuffings, an artful arrangement of bran muffins in clear plastic tins. "I always tell him, *enough* with the fancy displays!"

"I'm sorry, I'm so sorry," I sputtered on repeat, unhinging my white knuckled grip on my cart and attempting to bend over to help pick everything up.

The kind butcher stopped me before my fingertips could reach my knees.

"Just go, honey, just go," and she offered me a pretzel.

Generally in life you have three options: Lead, follow, or get out of the way.

I ate that pretzel, and got the heck out of the way.

Love,
Mom

CARROTS.

Thursday, July 8, 2010

Dear Babies,

I feel you kicking like crazy now! Both of you! Four limbs, twenty fingers, twenty toes!

This is insane!

I'll feel one of you down by my belly button and at the same time one up by my ribs. Sometimes I can follow the route of one of you, like you are going for swim, a goldfish making the rounds in his bowl.

I always loved parties and it makes me happy to know you're throwing one in here. Not only can I feel you but I can *see* you. Last night this perfect little hard round ball visibly popped up on my right side, like someone had screwed in a light bulb just beneath the surface of my skin. Maybe it was one of your heads, or even better, one of your little behinds.

Wow...

This is *happening.*

And I am just so excited...

I just can't wait to hold you.

Love,
Mom

Friday, July 9, 2010

Dear Babies,

Even though it was a little rainy out, I went for a walk around the reservoir.

I saw a jet black swan dive his whole body underneath the water and disappear beneath the murky surface. . .

When I got home I found an old journal stuck in a bottom drawer of my desk. Starting to go into "toss it or pack it" mode, I decided to stick it back in its rightful place up in a cardboard box on the top shelf of the bedroom closet, where other such "sentimental" items are stored. Trying to adhere to doctor's orders of avoiding heavy lifting, I nudged the box with my elbow until it fell to the floor with a thud. I sat with it straddled in my feet. I got so lost in this little box of moments. . . *reading old Valentine's Day cards from when your dad and I were dating. Christmas and birthday cards from my grandparents. Oh, to see their handwriting. I rubbed my hands over their words.* "Love, Pop." There was a note from my first boss wishing me well when she retired from her post at *More* magazine, forecasting my bright future. I wondered what she was doing now. . . she loved kayaking, didn't she?

You see there's all this stuff that happens in life, babies, and then there's the stuff that lives on beneath the surface. A memory we keep in our back pockets for when we need it, when we're sad, or lonely, or feeling reflective on a rainy day.

So much is going to happen in your lives.

You're going to meet so many people.

There's this saying I like: The mind forgets but the heart remembers.

And what it doesn't, you can always keep tucked away in a cardboard box.

Love,
Mom

Monday, July 12, 2010

Dear Babies,

I went into a Duane Reade today to buy deodorant. Seventy dollars later, I walked out with deodorant, face wash, sunscreen, organic coconut scented shampoo, black hair bands, and a canister of yogurt covered pretzels.

"Stuff" seems to be the theme these days as I sit here compiling this monster excel sheet of "stuff" I'm told we "need" for you guys to "live." We "need" crib bibs. And sheet savers. And if you're boys, these things called—wait for it— PeePee TeePees. (I swear).

We need to invent a baby product, fast.

I spent the whole weekend doing research for this, and not for safety standards or "best" brands people have recommended, *please*. I can count the number of times I've held a newborn on my right hand. I don't need your excel sheets of what's best, people. I need you to literally tell me what these baby products are. *A sleep sack? A swaddle me with Velcro? A sleep positioner?* Daylight Saving Time used to be the most confusing thing on the planet. Now, it's baby clothing, which is called "layette" in Momese.

Moms use the words t-shirts, undershirts and onesies all interchangeably. I mean, aren't they clearly three different things? Even you guys will be able to tell the difference between something that hits at your waist or snaps *beneath your crotch* like Nacho Libre.

Here's an example of a head-banging conversation between me and a mom:

ME: "How many t-shirts do I need?"

MOM: "Three packages."

ME: "Three, okay. What about onesies?"

MOM: "Onesies are t-shirts. You'll use the t-shirts until the umbilical cord falls off, then the onesies."

ME: "Right, okay, so how many do I need?"

MOM: "Three packages."

ME: "Three packs of t-shirts or three packs of onesies?"

Why is this so confusing? Are they so sleep-deprived that it all becomes a blur?

(Don't answer that.)

To add to the confusion, everyone has an opinion. Everyone has life-threatening do's and don'ts. Everyone has old crap they want to give me. "Your baby will be hot." "Your baby will be cold." "Your babies will be small." "Your babies will be big."

I can't listen to everyone, babies.

From now on it's just you and you and me, and the probably stupid things I decide to buy for you. Clothes with monkeys on them you will look back on in photos and cringe at with your bad haircuts, *thanks, Mom.*

If I go overboard buying deodorant, then I'm sure to go overboard when shopping for two newborns, and that's that.

Besides, monkeys are fun.

Love,
Mom

Tuesday, July 13, 2010

Dear Babies,

The following is an email I received today from Pampers.
com:

Hello, Amy!

*You are now in Week 22 of your pregnancy, and there are
exciting things to come for you and your baby!*

—Hemorrhoids

—Hello in There

—Notice a change in your hair?

I'm sorry, just what is exciting about hemorrhoids?

What is exciting is that I finally took care of that line of
hair I had going from here to here (use your imagination).
I know you can't tell from the inside, but from the outside,
wow, what a sight to behold. I am as taut, white and hairless
as a volleyball.

Love,
Mom

SPAGHETTI SQUASH.

Thursday, July 15, 2010

Dear Babies,

It's freezing.

Within minutes of finishing three slices of pizza yesterday for lunch I was asked what I wanted for dinner.

There was a near full-on battle at the house this morning over who likes Panera bread—YOU LOVE IT! NO, *YOU* LOVE IT! NO, *YOU* LOVE IT!

And, my choice of blue as a "gender neutral" color has become controversial, sparking digs on my behalf about dressing you guys like Shiloh Jolie-Pitt.

You guessed it: We're at Nanny and Grumpah's with Auntie Krissy for the weekend, where the air-conditioning is always blasting, where the fights are ridiculous, where we always talk about food.

Growing up this house was the food house. The "good junk food" house where all of my friends would gather to eat. Picture us on a TV sitcom with the plucky next door neighbor barging in uninvited, opening up the kitchen cabinets, squawking "got anything to eat?" (Or come your time will family sitcoms be completely extinct, wiped out by reality television? *The Bachelor 115,275: Still Looking, After All These Years. . .*) It got to the point when I would wonder *do my friends like me, or my mom's chicken cutlets?*

I never understood how we'd go out "driving around" for the night and they'd say they were hungry. That they hadn't eaten dinner. They'd look at me like I was the freak when I wouldn't order anything. *How can you not, we're at Kenny Rogers' Roasters?* If I hadn't just completed a home-cooked three course meal (every meal begins with pasta, even Thanksgiving, because nothing says, "let's kick off a turkey feast" like lasagna!), I knew there would be one waiting for me on the kitchen counter, wrapped in saran wrap ready to be reheated when I got home.

I used to be embarrassed by all of this. I dreaded lunchtime in the cafeteria when the other kids would unwrap sandwich bags of neat little triangles of turkey and cheese, and there I'd be, slowly uncoiling a tin foiled club of chicken parmesan so big it took two hands to bite. When I got to school my freshmen year of college in State College, PA I was like oh my God, what is this thing called *ranch*? I only ate Italian dressing growing up, and not even real "Italian," that comes in a bottle and has tiny flecks of seasoning in it, but home-mixed oil and vinegar my family called Italian. Imagine my surprise meeting people who actually ate Spaghetti O's. Chef Boyardee. Tomato sauce that comes *{gasp}* pre-made in a jar.

Food stories about the family could go on and on. There are all the Christmas Eves with the Seven Fishes sitting around a long table in Maga's basement shouting *pass the gal-uh-mah!* (Translated: calamari.) Maga is not just the matriarch of the family, she is a rare culinary MacGyver. Go on, give her breadcrumb, egg and an onion. She can whip up anything delicious in minutes.

My parents may have of done some things wrong. Grumpah trusted me to cover my eyes when watching television with him. Yeah, okay. *Thanks for* Nightmare on Elm Street *at age five!* But they did a lot of things right. We ate meals together as a family. Before I left the dinner table I would have to ask, may I be excused?

The things that drive you crazy about our family may be the things you grow up to love the most.

So embarrassing, you'll say at age 16.
At 30, so fondly, *so us...*
See you in the kitchen.

Love,
Mom

Monday, July 19, 2010

Dear Babies,

The days are flying by now. I look at the clock and see it's eight p.m. already and I sincerely wonder, *where did the time go?*

People said this would happen, especially once we passed the halfway mark, that it all would go by so fast. . .

Normally remarks like "good thing you're not working!" would grate on me as I'd be up sleepless nights at my laptop with my hands on my head staring at that damn blinking cursor, but these days, it's true. Aside from these letters, I'm not writing. I haven't written a word in three days. I am in full-on "nesting" mode. A stack of paint swatches for your nursery is by my side. I keep holding them up against your bedding, staring at them, walking closer, stepping back, contemplating the difference between Salty Tear and Tropical Pool.

I feel like I am playing house, babies, only this is real. This is very, very real.

The utter excitement about meeting you guys, like nothing I've ever experienced before, *is real.*

The excitement to move into our new home and start putting these magazine tears and paint swatches to work, is real.

And with that, so is the terror. The old gnawing fear that because things are going so well something bad is waiting to happen.

(Some people never feel they deserve happiness, babies. It is a terrible way to go through life.)

I'm trying to stay positive.

I'm trying to keep things light.

I'm staring at these little blue rectangles, getting lost in a world where the degree of green is the most important thing.

Salty tear? Tropical pool??

I pass the time.

It's all I can do.

Love,
Mom

Tuesday, July 20, 2010

Dear Babies,

I received another random email today from Pampers.
com which is making me wonder if I signed up for
something?

It began the same as last week's:

Hello, Amy!

*You are now in Week 23 of your pregnancy, and there are
exciting things to come for you and your baby!*

And this, too, had a very un-exciting sub-heading:

—*Empty Bladder.*

I mean, what the hell??? Peeing ten thousand times a day
is NOT exciting. Who writes this stuff? I'm convinced it's a
male. Young. Twenty-two right out of NYU. He wanted to be
a graphic designer for Deutsch but, "in this economy," had to
take the first job he could get. *Pampers.com.* His two geeky
roommates on St. Mark's Place make fun of him relentlessly.
As the bottom of the totem pole at work he got roped into taking on copy, too. Poor skinny Jason with thin wire-framed
glasses. His cords so slim, how does he get them over his feet.

Anyway, that same beacon of motherhood told me I
should be talking to you guys now. A lot. Or reading or singing. That it'll help you to recognize my voice later on.

So, *okay*. . .

{Clearing throat.}

"Hi!"

It feels strange.

I talk to myself all day anyway, isn't that enough?

No?

Well then, what should I talk to you guys about?

How great was it that Frank finally left The Bachelorette last night?—No, that won't do. You guys will be inevitably cooler than I am and won't care about "The Bachelorette."

It's six o'clock, should I push off work for yet another day and go back to looking at paint swatches? Little Pond? Caribbean Mist?—Or is that wrong, treating you guys like my personal Magic Eight ball seeking answers to my myriad indecisions?

How can your father open a drawer, see it has only shorts in it—since it is his 'shorts drawer'—and throw in a t-shirt? I don't understand. I may be a little anal but this should be a basic matching instinct. And the t-shirt drawer is right next to the shorts drawer. He was already bending over. Why not just open the shirt drawer and put the t-shirt back in its right place?—Okay, now I'm dragging you into my guy-from-*Sleeping-With-the-Enemy*-anal-insanity (those beautifully aligned soup cans!) and ranting needlessly about your father. Bad example. Sorry.

Sometimes when I'm out walking I put on the song "Baby Mine" from the *Beaches* soundtrack. When I show you this movie one day you'll see how truly masochistic this is, treading in such emotional territory for a hormonal pregnant woman.

baby mine, don't you cry
baby mine, dry your eyes
rest your head close to my heart
never to part, baby of mine

Sometimes when you don't know what to say, there's the perfect song. . .

I love you, babies of mine.

Love,
Mom

MANGOES.

Wednesday, July 21, 2010

Dear Babies,

Lunch with the girls. . . Seriously, every pizza should be sprinkled with truffle oil. And one of the best perks of being pregnant is that you always get to take home the leftovers.

So You Think You Can Dance is on tonight. . .

Your father just got home early. . .

It's 5:30 p.m. and I am already in my pajamas. . .

Twenty-three weeks today and you guys are the size of mangoes, and I do love me some mangoes.

Wow, what a day.

Love,
Mom

Friday, July 23, 2010

Dear Babies,

It's 1:30 p.m. on a rainy Friday afternoon and I am sitting with my chin in my fist, gazing out the window.

You'll love Fridays, babies. Rain or shine.

As stressful and dreaded as Mondays are, Fridays bring a sense of relief—*I made it!*—mixed with a sense of play. How great that we as a society leave our problems, our homework, our looming deadlines aside for two whole days and enjoy this thing called the weekend.

Maybe Friday will be pizza night. Maybe pizza and a movie. Maybe we'll meet your father with roadie cups at the door when he gets home from the train and walk down to the beach (you lucky ducks, getting to grow up in a town so close to the water).

Fridays bring a sense of promise. Maybe tomorrow you will wake up early and get back to the gym, you haven't been all week. Clean out the closets. Go out on Saturday night and meet the man of your dreams. Maybe next week will be better than the one before.

Maybe...

Love,
Mom

Monday, July 26, 2010

Dear Babies,

The house is freezing cold. . .

This morning, over a breakfast of scrambled eggs and home fries with triangles of buttered toast, there was a full-out debate over what we were having for dinner—flounder rolled with spinach and breadcrumbs, or pasta with marinara sauce—which was a waste of time since we all knew we would end up with both.

Grumpah set off mass hysteria when he dumped a bucket of chemicals into the pool while I was floating around in it like Baby Beluga. . .

{Sigh.}

You guessed it, we're back at Nanny's. Your dad is in LA for work and was worried about me being alone. Because it's so peaceful here. Right.

Last night at a party he met Mary Murphy from *So You Think You Can Dance*. He sent a video of her putting me and both of you on her "hot tomale train," complete with one of her signature earsplitting "who-hoo's!"

"Did you get video?" he called to ask, like this was normal.

Oh, sure. I can't touch my toes. Grumpah is blasting *Mothra*, a 1962 Japanese science-fiction movie dubbed so horribly I'm about to lose my mind (then ten-seconds later, you would see my lips move).

"Yes, very funny," I said, like it *was* normal, watching a woman I see on television every Tuesday night reference me and my unborn children. All par for the course.

Time to go stare at the ceiling.

AKA, time for bed.

Love,
Mom

Tuesday, July 27, 2010

Dear Babies,

We are twenty-four weeks tomorrow. You guys will be ears of corn in the middle of summer, how apropos.

I write this to you from my childhood bed under four comforters. It's almost midnight and I can't sleep, shocker. It's just like the old days of me in the dark writing in a journal, except totally different.

We have another doctor's appointment tomorrow. I was right, the fact that I can feel you guys moving and kicking hasn't changed a thing, I'm still as nervous as ever. *I just want to hear two heartbeats, and that everything is okay.*

Maybe I'll read one of those parenting books piling up and collecting dust on my bedside table. *Ferberizing vs. Attachment Parenting? Feed/wake/sleep schedules? The magical five s's to soothe a crying baby? Am I preparing for motherhood or training to become a sleep-inducing ninja with the touch of my hand?* This should knock me out in no time...

Love,
Mom

EARS OF CORN.

Wednesday, July 28, 2010

Dear Babies,

Everything went well at our appointment. Baby A, you are head down and ready to go. Baby B, as of now you're breach, poised to come into the world ass first. Our doctor said there's plenty of time for you to keep spinning around and "right" yourself. I asked her, "what about me?" as in, is *there still time for me to right my ass-backward self in this world?* She looked at me and blinked.

Auntie Krissy came with me and afterward we went out to lunch and got massages and facials. Sounds nice, right? But no one knows you like a sibling, babies. When Auntie Krissy saw me coming out of my massage room, emerging pink faced with my hair disheveled like Doc from *Back to the Future*, she started laughing hysterically. I started laughing, too. She knew I didn't enjoy it. That I was just not comfortable lying there like a washed-up giant squid, all lubed. She knows my mind cannot calm down enough to enjoy such things of "relaxation." That I'm too "in it," present in the room, to not think about what's going on around me. *How weird is it that they are playing swanky hotel lounge music? Where is the Buddha chanting and the chimes? I feel like a well coiffed man in a slim-cut Dolce & Gabbana suit should be taking me to my room and handing me a bellini.* I wished that were happening. Instead. . . I was face down with my belly wedged into a crater of a pillow. My nose was itchy. If I didn't shift my neck and swallow I would release a strand of drool Turner and Hooch-style to the floor. No matter how great a foot rub it was, I still had two kicking babies inside of me going Rocky on my ribs and a tad bit o' gas from the spicy curly fries at lunch. (Sorry, TMI.)

We cackled walking out together thinking of another person who also notoriously doesn't enjoy a good rub down: Our mother.

Maybe we inherit more than we think.

Love,
Mom

Friday, July 30, 2010

Dear Babies,

Okay, now Pampers.com is really stretching it. I just got the following email from them:

Hello Amy,

Now that you're in your sixth month-and obviously preg-nant-you're probably thinking more about caring for that little one growing inside you.

At first glance this seemed okay, but then I went back and dissected and analyzed (because if you are girls, this will be your specialty):

1.) I'm actually almost done with my sixth month, I start seven months on Wednesday.

2.) I'd say that the first three months of nausea and dry heaving until I burst the capillaries on my face made it pretty obvious I was pregnant to me.

3.) *Now* I'm probably thinking about caring for you guys? Oh, okay. *NOW* I'm thinking about you guys, as opposed to the past six months when it's been party central, I've really been stringing up the lights over here, footloose and fancy free.

Funny stuff.

Shark Week starts on Sunday.

Your father says he doesn't get it. *What's the big deal? There are shark shows on all the time!* But I grew up watching Shark Week. After a long day of swimming in the pool with my cousins, we'd come in, shower, get in our pajamas, turn on the air conditioning—which was a treat in itself, trust me, having to beg Grumpah to let us put it on, the nights when he said no camping out in front of the living room windows in hopes of catching a breeze. . .

It's the experience of things.

It's the memories.

Love,
Mom

Monday, August 2, 2010

Dear Babies,

The phrase of the day is "holy crap."

As in, *holy crap*, I can't believe it's August already!

That I ate an entire baguette, with a whole avocado and innumerable slices of swiss cheese!

That I started hysterically crying as I was walking out of Staples carrying a paper shredder when a classical version of "Rock-A-Bye Baby" started playing on my iPod!

Holy crap, *it's four o'clock already. . .*

And we are moving in six weeks!

And there is so much to do!

And I still haven't taken off my sneakers from my morning walk because I cannot reach my feet!

Holy crap, I am so excited for Christmas. I saw it on an episode of *Mad Men* last night. Joanie in her holiday sweater. Your father calls me a "drunken elf" because I get so excited during the holiday season (which starts here on Thanksgiving Eve, not that I'm counting down or anything).

Holy crap, *you are going to be here for Thanksgiving. . .*

And Christmas. . .

I can't wait to listen to holiday music with you guys, delirious at three a.m. feedings, maybe by the glow of a dimly lit Christmas tree. "Silent Night." "Have Yourself a Merry Little Christmas." (Bing Crosby's a cappella version always makes me cry.)

I can't imagine my heart being any fuller with love for you than it is right now.

I can't imagine...

But holy crap, it will be.

Love,
Mom

Tuesday, August 3, 2010

Dear Babies,

I met a woman at the gym this morning who is due next week and we, at seven months, were twice her size.

{High five.}

{High five.}

By the way, I had no idea what the taxi driver was saying before either. That certainly was not English.

I love having someone to commiserate with over such things. . .

Like last night, with all the kicking, it was clear you, too, found *The Bachelorette* finale as torturous as I did. On top of each mention of the word "journey" I wanted to vomit over Roberto's *mi amor*'s. *Thank you very much-o Mr.-o Robert-o,* I quipped out loud. One of you must have thought that was funny. A foot or a knee or something came sprouting up like a little mushroom. *Good one, Mom!*

Okay, back to paper shredding. How fun is our new shredder? Why didn't we get one of these sooner? Your father is going to come home not to an apartment but to me sitting up like a cumbersome polar bear in a mound of confetti.

Love,
Mom

RUTABAGAS.

Wednesday, August 4, 2010

Dear Babies,

So, this would have previously been a note to self ("Self:") but now I have you two to inherit my pearls of wisdom.

Babies:

Don't walk past a six-foot standing fan with an open recycling pail full of a million little pieces of shredded paper.

As soon as I finish picking this white confetti snow out of my hair, ears, lips, and cleavage (think Joe Pesci in *Home Alone* when he gets blasted with down feathers while coated in honey), I will get dressed so we can go meet your father for dinner.

Five Napkin Burger.

French onion soup. Pickles. Macaroni and cheese. Onion rings. Bring it on.

Happy twenty-five weeks.

Love,
Mom

Thursday, August 5, 2010

Dear Babies,

I ate a whole pineapple, then keeled over in pain, popped a million papaya pills (they work way better than Tums), and fell asleep on the couch.

Everyone says how great it is that I eat so much fruit.

I don't think they really consider the ramifications of this.

I am Al Bundy, babies.

I'm so sorry.

Love,
Mom

Friday, August 6, 2010

Dear Babies,

In case you felt a million eyes upon us as we were walking up and down Broadway, I can explain. . .

It all started when I ran out to buy a Vera Bradley duffle bag for Nanny for her birthday this weekend.

Not expecting to be out long, I threw on a short cotton sundress that used to be "blousy" and a pair of so-cheesy-but-so-comfy spongy flip-flops. (They have rhinestones.) On my way out I grabbed my knee-high lace-up boots and threw them into a Bloomingdale's shopping bag thinking I better do something about that duck-like squeaking that haunted me all winter, because that had to get done today, in August. Before I walked out the door I caught a glimpse of myself in the mirror and saw that the dress, already too tight and too short, looked even shorter and tighter when paired with the big, foamy sandals. (With the rhinestones.) My hair was in a high pony. The only thing missing was a scrunchie.

By the time I got to the corner my feet already hurt. The clunky bag was banging into my bare calves with each step. I got stuck at the light with a Hasidic couple and their eight small children. They were all clad in black turtlenecks and pants or thick long skirts with black tights underneath. Black sneakers. Yet I was the one profusely sweating. I began twisting my ponytail into a coil and wiping the sweat that was dripping off the back of my neck with my hand. I looked at the children. They looked at me. I was as close to the water scene in *Flashdance* as they were ever going to get.

When I got to the shoe place one block away the bag felt so heavy I couldn't wait to drop it off. But there I learned they couldn't do anything for me. The quacking duck was internal. *Dammit.* Not only would I be squawking through next winter, but I would have to heave the monstrous bag back onto my shoulder. I took a deep breath and slid it up to my elbow accepting my fate.

When I got to the next store to buy my mother's gift, I was told they had no more Vera Bradley bags.

Son of a!

Not willing to admit defeat, I meandered around the home section determined to buy *something,* and ended up with a clear plastic shower cap covered with fluorescent pink flamingoes. I threw that into the growing-heavier-by-the-minute bag and left, deciding Nanny's gift would have to wait. I couldn't carry it anymore, the next stop would have to be home...

Until I saw the sign across the street calling to me like a beacon in the night.

—*H&H Bagels.*—

Suddenly, I had to have a bagel.

Plain and heated up in the microwave for 30 seconds.

(Had to.)

I justified the stop, thinking I could get bagels for tomorrow morning, thereby helping your father and I get out the door faster to make our ferry to Fire Island. *I'd be saving us time! I'd be a hero!* A real Nelson Mandela.

I stepped inside...

Oh, the smell of fresh baked bagels...

I took another step and quickly realized my dream was a nightmare.

No A.C.

It was so friggin' hot in there.

Only working ovens and ten thousand people and apparently no cashiers.

Great.

Still, in the name of little circles of goodness I mean getting us to Fire Island on time, *I would suffer.* I thought of Indiana Jones on a mission. I likened my battle with heat and encroaching sweaty-people to Indie's quest for the Holy Grail. Now I know, my own personal Holy Grail is carbohydrates with scallion cream cheese.

Within minutes I was melting, Jack Frost roasting on an open fire. Sweat was not only dripping down my forehead and my face but also my back and bare glistening legs and onto my spongy shoes with a splat.

I coiled my ponytail onto my head yet again and began fanning myself with the tub of scallion cream cheese I'd grabbed from the fridge. *Can I fit in there? Can I??* I'd thought in that split second the icy door was cracked.

The woman behind me tried to bond, complaining about the huge line, the extreme heat, "what, is everyone who works here on coffee break?" But it was too hot for chit-chat. I smiled meekly and then turned around, giving her a nice view of the sweat beads sliding down my neck, little Olympians on the luge. I stood still, impatiently waiting my turn.

Finally, I got a dozen bagels, the tub of cream cheese, and threw *that* into the already two-ton bag.

I contemplated eating a bagel on the final stretch home, only it was too much effort to reach down and pull one out of the bag within a bag. So I stopped into Tasti Delight and got a chocolate peanut-butter milkshake instead. Obviously.

Just as I put the pink straw to my lips I felt the bottom of the bag give out. *Come on, we're so close!* I then proceeded to limp the rest of the way home, resting the ripping bag on my hip with one hand, holding my milkshake in the other, my dress riding further and further up with each step. . .

Sometimes the littlest task can feel like walking through fire. You'll remember you have to stop at the dry cleaners after work and groan that's *torture. All you want to do is go home, take these damn shoes off, and feast.* Daily life can be tough, babies. But remember, very often it's you marching yourself into these situations. Just as easily, you can march yourself out. Don't make things harder than they need to be.

Life is the result of the choices we make.

As Indie was told on his search for the Holy Grail, *choose wisely.*

Love,
Mom

Monday, August 9, 2010

Dear Babies,

If you can feel the rumblings of my stomach, hear outside noises, sense light, then you must be able to feel the heaviness of my heart.

Mickey, Nanny and Grumpah's dog, our dog, the "coffee table" who was the fourth person to hear the wonderful news of your arrival, *remember?* He died this morning. After a year-long battle with lymphoma he suffered a rapid deterioration this past weekend and had to be put to sleep.

We all knew it was coming.

We looked into his sad, brown eyes and saw his suffering, his fear. We knew it was the right and the only thing to do.

"Humane," as people who don't know what to say will say.

Still, no matter how strong and prepared you think you are, nothing can ease the hurt of losing a pet.

Your father came home from work today to take me to lunch. Over tater tots and lemonade at Big Daddy's he said that this was why he didn't think he could ever get a dog.

"No," I told him emphatically, "No! All the years of joy and unconditional love they bring outweigh all of this."

And that's what I want you to remember, babies. That all the good times and memories of a life outweigh all the bad.

Mickey is up there right now looking down on us, relieved that Nanny doesn't have to be home to mash up a baked potato for him anymore, boil him chicken, sneak him medicine into rolled up slices of American cheese. He is bonding with Brandon, my old dog, the one that I grew up with, who is probably ribbing him for not being "bad enough."—*What do you mean, you didn't bark at fresh loaves of Italian bread on the table until they gave in? I did!*—Maybe he is even with Poppy, they were together here for such a short time. Poppy used to tease him and call him a cat. Mickey had some sauce to him. I picture him up there walking over to Pop, grinning and saying *meow.*

No matter where he is or what he is doing, I know he is looking out for us. That he did this for us knowing he wouldn't make it through the fall so Nanny could be free to focus on you guys, and help us. . .

Last year on August 13th your father and I had our first failed fertility treatment. My heart was broken and I cried for days while Mickey sat quietly at my feet.

Mimi tried to comfort me by reminding me in her warm Southern drawl that the hurt would pass.

—*Hon-nay, this time next year we'll all be worrying about something else. . .* —

This year on August 13th I am getting a pregnancy ultrasound for not one but two healthy babies.

I am not worrying this time.

I am comforted knowing we have another angel up there looking out for us. The kindest kind. The innocent.

Love,
Mom

Tuesday, August 10, 2010

Dear Babies,

There's this story about the weakness of man, something about walking into a cave and seeing this giant red button that says "END OF THE WORLD, DO NOT PRESS!" And then, well...

So I got my weekly ridiculous email from Pampers.com today:

Hello Amy,

You are now in Week 26 of your pregnancy, and there are exciting things to come for both you and your baby!

—Heartburn

—Moisturizing

—Bleeding Gums

In other words:

—A chest-clenching nightly inferno.

—Tight, itchy skin stretched to the max.

—Looking like a *Twilight* cast-member reject every morning when I brush my teeth.

Exciting!

In the mood to futz around with "baby stuff"online, but not read any more of that, I flipped through a similar email I'd gotten from Babycenter.com.

This week you will be the size of English hothouse cucumbers. Who knew.

In the top right corner of an article I was reading on anemia (you know, light reading), I saw this eye-catching link.

"3D animated video about the stages of labor and birth!" flashed a triangular button over a cartoon drawing of a baby's pink head turned upside down in a womb.

Click me! Click me! Click me!

("END OF WORLD, DO NOT PRESS!")

I clicked. . .

OH, MY GOD, BABIES!!!!! WHAT WAS I THINKING!!! THERE WAS NO NEED FOR ME TO SEE THOSE THINGS!!! THERE IS NO NEED FOR ANYONE TO EVER SEE THOSE THINGS!!! DOCTORS, FOR THE LOVE OF PETE (btw, who's Pete?), KEEP IT TO YOURSELVES!!!

I've had women ask me, "So, what's your birth plan?" I've tossed this off, thinking, what do you mean, like I have a choice in the matter? *I'll have a grande non-fat latte and a vaginal birth, please.* "To get them out," I respond jokingly, prompting a few laughs. *Ha, ha, fluffy pregnant girl who looks like a panda is being funny and cute!* But now more than ever, after seeing that eye-sore of a video, I am not being funny, nor cute.

Damn right that's my birth plan.

Do what you gotta do down there. Just GET. THEM. OUT.

Love,
Mom

ENGLISH HOTHOUSE CUCUMBERS.

Wednesday, August 11, 2010

Dear Babies,

It's Wednesday, August 11th, an otherwise ordinary day except that today I have peed more than on any other day.

(This really must be some kind of a record.)

It also is the day I am declaring I have officially lost all shame.

When you're pregnant, it doesn't matter what you *wear*. You can throw style to the wind (or in this case, public flatulence) because nobody cares about things like visible panty lines or blatant bra straps *when you have an alien growth protruding from your stomach.*

We leave for vacation on Saturday, Montauk for a week and a half. Normally I would have gone to Anthropologie to pick up cute new pajamas and maybe a whimsical sundress or two, but today I went to Filene's Basement.

I stood in front of a mirror in the middle of the "intimate apparel" section with a pile of prospects on the floor beside me and tried on everything, right there, on top of my clothes.

A bathrobe that could wrap around my midriff, and therefore also a sub-zero fridge. . . (Check!)

A racerback cotton tank top to sleep in, size XL. . . (Check!)

A silky, frilly, Oscar de la Renta nightgown that looks like it belonged on a hook on the back of a door in Miss Hannigan's bathroom. . . (Ch—oh, no thanks.)

And the clincher, the classiest of classy, two white strapless bras. (I couldn't decide between a C cup or a D, oh how I've waited my whole life for such a dilemma!)

Yes, babies, I tried on bras right on top of my tight red cotton sundress surrounded by shoppers and workers in the middle of the downstairs level of Filene's Basement. I fully cinched the back, squeezed my boobs in, did the proverbial "lift up" with my hands, stood back, tilted my head, examined, as if I were in the confines of my bedroom. A male salesman made eye contact with me in the mirror from behind, dropped his head and quickly looked away.

Today is Wednesday, August 11th. Of these days of new normals, an ordinary day indeed.

Love,
Mom

Thursday, August 12, 2010

Dear Babies,

Here are things I am not going to miss about the city when we leave:

1.) Having to walk everywhere in the rain, stepping into dark, mystery puddles at curbs and splatting dirty water up onto my bare calves.

2.) Seeing human feces in the subway station (it was too large to be canine, too small to be horse).

3.) Encountering a blaring mariachi band on the downtown 1 train each morning on my way to work when I just want to be tired, when I'm not ready to see humans yet, when I want to keep my head down in a book but no—*La Cucaracha!*

4.) Sharing the laundry room and washing machines with strangers. (Who is still using mothballs, WHO?!)

5.) Having to make small talk with these strangers as I load and unload the machines. I don't want to talk about the weather. Ever. Especially not in a basement laundry room that feels like *hey this would be a good place for the guy from* Saw *to set up shop* and I'm not wearing a bra.

6.) Rolling over a long-dead cockroach with my laundry cart.

7.) Seeing an obese, scruffy man sitting in front of the Gap in the rain with a smeared cardboard sign that says "Out of work, Out of Luck, Please Help." My heart can't take not helping these guys. They're likely drug-addicted maniacs, but still.

That's it for now. . .

Feel free to remind me of this list when you hear me and your father wax poetic on how much we miss the city.

(Though the mariachi band was really good, I'm not gonna lie.)

Love,
Mom

Friday, August 13, 2010

Dear Babies,

I had my diabetes test today. Everyone talked about the syrup I would have to take, *the syrup!* But I thought it was nothing. I literally gulped it down in two sips. *I went to Penn State*, I boasted to the respectable nurse practitioner wiping the sticky corners of my mouth. For some reason, she seemed unimpressed by my frat-boy chugging skills. Your father rolled his eyes at me. *"Really?"*

Afterward we had our regular doctor's appointment and ultrasound upstairs. Your dad and I marveled over how big you are getting, almost two and a half pounds each! How strong your two hearts were beating. How bored you guys must be. Baby A, you kept fiddling with your ear.

On the way home I sat in the backseat of a taxi cruising down Riverside Drive with the window down just about so, fresh air grazing the top of my forehead. The late afternoon sun was casting an amber glow on the giant speckled sycamore trees lining the West Side highway. People were out in the park, some with dogs, teens in baseball uniforms, the elderly getting walked in their wheelchairs, babies pushed in strollers.

With my hair slightly blowing, I closed my eyes and said, *Thank you, God, thank you. . .*

Love,
Mom

Tuesday, August 24th, 2010

Dear Babies,

After ten days at the beach we are back.

Back to life...

Back to reality...

Back to routine, which unfortunately for us includes watching the two-hour mind suck that is *Bachelor Pad*.

When you get older and have a job, step outside and take a lunch break.

If you live in the city take a road trip and get out for a day, for a weekend, if you can.

Use up every single one of your allotted vacation days. (My first job, including sick days, allotted a whopping five.)

If you go away to college, please, come home. Not because of selfish reasons, like that I miss you already just thinking about this, but because there's something magical about going away, and then coming home.

It makes you appreciate everything you have so much more.

The comfort of your own bed.

The sight of your razor in the shower.

The bakery on your corner, the fruit stand guy, the Chinese take-out place, the way the trees form sweeping arches over your block...

Home.

Growing up there was this sign that hung next to the steps heading down to our basement. It said in red stenciled paint on a scalloped wooden wreath, "home is where you hang your heart," with this little dangling heart in the center.

. . . We start our third trimester tomorrow.

Aside from finding out I'm anemic last week ("Your sugar is fine! But your iron is low," which is to be expected of a quasi-vegetarian pregnant with twins, I mean how much more spinach can I eat?) what a remarkable ride this has been.

We're getting close, babies.

You're on your way home.

Love,
Mom

HEADS OF CAULIFLOWER.
(*BIG*)

200

Wednesday, August 25, 2010

Dear Babies,

At the doctor's office today I learned that since you guys are slightly ginormous—in the 68th percentile for size, bigger than single babies at this point, Godzilla-size for twins—we're going back for another ultrasound in three weeks rather than four. Then probably one or two weeks after that. Then, well, she said maybe another at thirty-four weeks, "if you're still pregnant by then."

Holy. . . crap.

I called your dad. He was at a lunch. I told him to have a drink. And then another. He told me to hurry up and schedule the nursery furniture for delivery.

Back at the ranch (our one bedroom apartment) I began to prep for our move.

I scheduled your crib delivery. (Priority)

I called our church and told them I was moving and to stop sending envelopes. (Not priority)

I sweated through my shorts (sorry) looking at a friend's registry, stressing over what to send her as a gift for her wedding I cannot attend. This wedding is in October. (Not priority)

I looked up Long Island cleaning companies to clean the house before we move in. (Priority)

"Welcome to Aftermath, Inc," one site began.

We specialize in cleanup services in the aftermath of:
-Homicide/murder and other violent crimes
-Suicide, suicide attempts and self-inflicted wounds
-Unattended deaths and decomposition/odor removal
-Vehicle blood clean-up
-Hoarding and filth

-*Tear gas remediation*
-*Methamphetamine labs*
I should be in a state of panic right now.

Instead here I sit with my feet up on my desk, eating Tate's dark-chocolate chip cookies, crafting different voice-mails for the above company in my mind.

Press 1 if you've just committed a murder.

Press 2 if your meth lab just burst into flames.

Press 3 if you're a hoarder, and congratulations on finding the phone...

Love,
Mom

Thursday, August 26th, 2010

Dear Babies,

Today was a prime example of sucking it up and marching into a situation you know is going to be a nightmare because you know it's something you just have to do.

When I stood in front of 135 W. 70th Street, Suite 1L, I could not believe the sight before me.

A brassy door, thick and gleaming gold like the entryway to Oz, engraved with the store name in a circle in the center:

Upper Breast Side

I pulled it open, struggling with the weight, and walked through. . .

"Hello! Would you like some chocolate? Some fresh peach-strawberry water?" the chipper receptionist sang, already up on her feet to pour me an ice cold drink. "Is this your first time here?"

"Yes, yes, and YES!" I beamed back, matching her cheeriness as I took a seat on the plush waiting room couch with my delicious beverage amid an assortment of plush toys, sheep and giraffes, and folded sherpa baby blankets.

I sighed, looking around, then said out loud, "I love it here!"

The ray of sunshine pampering me smiled warmly, pleased.

Then a voice called from the back.

"Amy? Fran will see you now, right behind the curtain. . . "

It really is like Oz!

I pushed through the zebra print fabric and crossed over to the other side. . .

"Are you Fran?" I said timidly to a woman who was Bea Arthur's clone, and may or may not have fit the late Miss Arthur for her very first training bra.

She dipped her dark framed sliver of glasses at me, "*Yeeees...*"

"Oh! Okay! I'm Amy!" I continued in a voice that couldn't have been higher if I'd just inhaled helium.

"*Yeeeees,*" she repeated, dipping the glasses lower, "how can I help you?"

I'd like a brain, a heart, some courage... "Oh! Okay! Well, I need a nursing bra, but I hate bras..."

And the glasses dipped even *lower.*

"So, I'm hoping to get some, nursing stuff—" and I pointed to the assortment of stacked cotton tank tops and stretchy shirts piled around the room with my chin.

"What's your pre-pregnancy bra size?" she interrupted, sliding her glasses back up the bridge of her nose with one push from her bony index finger.

"Uh, well, I don't really kno—

"—Bawl park fig-yah," she snapped, her paper thin patience vaporizing into the air. Before I could get out "34B" I was wrapped up in tape measure.

SNAP.

"What's your due date?"

"Um, well," I hemmed and hawed again, starting to explain how, since it's twins, we can't really know for sure because they'll probably come early...

"Sit down," she ordered.

I sat down onto a black velvet ottoman, squatting ass first like a sumo wrestler. I cleared my throat, as if that would mask the fact that I'd just crushed a few boxes of nude camisoles in my wake.

. . . Three-hundred and twelve dollars later, I walked out of Oz with three bras, three tank tops, a box of cold compress gel pads for my nipples, and a spinning head.

"Good-bye! Good luck! Do you want some more chocolate?" the ever-so-lovely receptionist called as I whizzed by. Sure, I realized, *they're so nice out here, literally sugar coating the nightmare in there.* I thought of the poor fish tricked out of its life by the promise of food.

At the corner I replayed the last conversation I'd had with Fran while flipping the outside of the bag that boasted the hot pink label "UPPER BREAST SIDE" to face the inside of my calf. A teen boy stood next to me. I did not want to deal with the glares.

— "You registered for Dr. Brown's bottles? Oh. No. Beverly recommends Playtex."

"Who?"

"Beverly. The Lactation Goddess? Here's her num-buh. Give her a cawl."—

I whipped out the crumbled piece of paper I'd shoved into my shopping bag and stared at a card that said "Bev" and a number.

Twins? You're going to need to rent a hospital-grade pump.

You're going to need storage bags.

Look at this {insert visual of dominatrix-looking bra here}, *you pump hands free. . .*

I don't know, babies.

Women in the Dark Ages didn't have cold compress gel pads for their nipples. Fancy boob stores on the manor. *Camelot's Cantaloupes.*

They didn't have Fran feeling them up while bitching about missing the 4:52 back home to Long Island.

They didn't need Bev.

Maybe I don't either.

Love,
Mom

Friday, August 27, 2010

Dear Babies,

I am sitting here at my desk staring at a breast pump like it is a UFO that just landed on my cornfield.

If I were a caveman, I would beat it with a stick to try to get it to work.

Since I don't have a stick, I might have to use my pencil.

What the hell am I doing, babies?

What... the hell... am I doing.

Love,
Mom

Monday, August 30, 2010

Dear Babies,

I am a mother, dammit.

I have everything under control.

I make informed decisions.

I remain cool under pressure.

I am a disciplinary figure.

. . . Oh come on, don't laugh!

I'm sorry I locked us out of the apartment today!

That other set of keys, they looked just like mine! If you could see them, you'd agree.

I know it really sucked sitting out there in the hallway on the dirty floor, sweating, having to pee, waiting for dad to come home from work to bail us out. I had all of our groceries with us, but everything required a fork. I contemplated biting into the wedge of jarlsburg, thinking of all the times I check my teeth in the elevator mirror, Earl on the security cameras had probably seen me do worse. But I didn't do it. *I am a beacon of exemplary behavior.*

. . . I brag about you already. ("So big!")

. . . When I say that I don't "love" being pregnant because I can't take the constant worry and sometimes feeling sick, I lie. I love placing my hands on my stomach. I love always having you with me. I love when your dad reaches over and presses his hands on me and delights over each pummel and kick. I love you two so much and I always will, no matter what.

After all, I am a mother.

Love,
Mom

Tuesday, August 31, 2010

Dear Babies,

Today is your cousin's first birthday.

So much happens in a year.

This time last year I was mustering the strength to sit in a maternity ward all day surrounded by the babies I so desperately longed for without breaking down and crying, and being able to show how genuinely happy I was for him to be born.

Today I sit rubbing my pregnant belly eating peanut butter straight from the jar.

I cannot walk down the street without taxis honking at me, either taking pity on my painfully slow waddle as I tackle crosswalks assuming I must need a ride, or saying hurry up, Shamu.

Men with not many teeth lurking in shadows in front of bodegas and drinking from brown paper bags make hush-toned predictions in my direction that I sometimes think might be true based on the criteria that they are 1.) crazy and 2.) old, like I've entered some voodoo cabin in the back-woods of New Orleans and not a deli under scaffolding on Amsterdam. "I'll tell you one thing, that right there be a boy. . ."

When I graduated college in 2001 I joined a group called ED2010. It posted daily job listings and industry news to help young fledglings like myself in magazine publishing achieve their "dream job" by the year 2010. A good way to see if you're on the right career path is to look at your bosses, *do you want their job?* While I saw I did not, I still chased after those listings. I wanted to be a writer, which at the time I thought meant feeling validated by working at a big-name magazine. (You really don't know half the things you think you do at 22.)

Today I realize—as clarity does come with age, babies, not just "old" age but any age, any time you can look back on an experience and see it objectively and learn from it—I don't need someone to tell me I'm a writer. I am one. I've always been one. I wrote the "Blackbeard Murders" in crayon when I was five. I'll always be one, the way someone is a pessimist, or is someone who simply does not eat peas.

. . . Funny how another role has popped up just in time for this 2010 deadline: Motherhood. I can't help but wonder, has this been the plan all along?

I really don't care for dream anything, babies. It cheapens things. Makes it all seem so Barbie. Dream house. Dream job. Dream man.

I do like thinking about the paths we take. The choices we make. The *hard things* we go through to get us to that big picture. Maybe we should see life like this:

Steps on a ladder, year after year.

Love,
Mom

BUTTERNUT SQUASH.

Thursday, September 2, 2010

Dear Babies,

We started week twenty-nine yesterday. Our doctor said you could be here around thirty-four or thirty-five. Math may not be my thing, but you don't need to be John Nash to figure out this means we're getting close.

I'd be freaking out right now if this heat hadn't sedated me. An official heat advisory has been issued urging small children and adults with disabilities not to go outside and to limit physical activity. Since I technically qualify as both, I will be adhering to the warning.

I'm like a warped vodka ad, loafing on the couch in nothing but a very long tank top in front of the A/C with a handheld fan, "Absolute Pregnant."

Love,
Mom

Friday, September 3, 2010

Dear Babies,

Your dad took off work today to tackle the daunting task of disconnecting all of our electronic stuff and wires in preparation for our move in two weeks.

Let me tell you, once when I was home alone with a cable repairman working in the apartment he took one look at all of our gadgets and wires and said to me, "Do you know you're married to Sup-ah Geek?"

"Yes, yes I do," I deadpanned at the time, but at this moment, standing in our living room amidst so many cable cords it's like the snake scene in *Raiders of the Lost Ark* ("SNAKES!"), Sup-ah Geek is no laughing matter.

Any minute now a woman should be arriving at our apartment to teach us infant CPR and child care and safety. This sounds like one of those things you see on a reality TV show where women are learning pole dancing in a neighbor's basement on a Tuesday night and you're like, there's no *way* they are just doing this, the show *must* be making them do this to have something to film. But oh no. I genuinely signed us up for this. I just scolded your father to straighten up and get ready to pay attention, to "show some respect to this woman who is coming into our home and preparing us for our children."

(Yes, I said that.)

(Verbatim.)

I guess with you guys arriving soon, I feel like I need to be doing *something*. So I'm buying things. I'm finally

214

reading those books. I'm taking classes. Let me practice putting a diaper on a doll, *please*...

I'm just getting nervous, that's all.

I guess I am Sup-ah Geek, too.

Love,
Mom

Tuesday, September 7, 2010

Dear Babies,

I'm not gonna lie, there are many days when I wake up and the first thought to enter my mind is, *Oy.*

Not so much, "Oy, I don't want to go to work today," but rather griping, *oy,* in response to the physicality of the day.

I think literally, *How am I going to get out of bed right now? How are we going to make it to the bathroom? To the kitchen? Shower? Sit at a desk all day in a chair?*

This third trimester of pregnancy is coinciding nicely with the waning days of summer, our days are getting shorter. The amount of functioning, productive hours I'm able to give are less and less.

But this morning I mustered all of the energy I had and swung out of bed genuinely enthused.

"It's all happening!" I thought, quoting *Almost Famous,* one of my favorite movies I may or may not have already quoted for you hundreds of times, each time promising that one day we'll watch it together. (If you're girls, we'll all want to be Penny Lane.)

We're on our way to a final walk-through of our new house tonight. (And, your dad doesn't know this yet, on the drive home we're stopping in Queens at Gyro Corner.)

Tomorrow, we close.

Work and paint, especially in your room, starts the end of this week.

As do the furniture deliveries, your nursery assembly, cleaning. . .

This time next week, we will officially *live* there, in a *house,* in the *suburbs.*

And before we know it, you guys will be living there with us, too, as a family.

Yes, it's all happening.

Love,
Mom

CABBAGES.

Wednesday, September 8, 2010

Dear Babies,

It's 10:00 p.m. and I'm utterly exhausted but I want to let you guys know that it is official:

We are home owners.

Today we closed on our house.

I sat in a conference room throughout the closing, signing things, hoping at any given moment a young assistant would enter offering a platter of mini-bagel sandwiches. (One didn't.)

On the drive out to the house after I sat in the car, quiet, looking out the window with my chin in my fist. (I was quite mad about the sandwiches.)

I sat in the kitchen on a folding chair your dad provided. "Sit," he ordered before darting off to go measure things.

"This is where the table will go," I thought as I sat alone. Me on a chair in a warm empty room, like a raisin plod into pudding.

As if pulled by a magnet, I rose and sauntered up the stairs.

The fourth one creaks, watch it.

I found myself in your vacant bedroom.

I ran my hand along the yellow wall, *this will soon be Harbor Fog,* then turned to slide my back down it until I reached the wood floor. Some dust bunnies blew.

And there I sat, barefoot and pregnant.

My elbows resting on my splayed open knees to allow room for my belly.

I closed my eyes and heard your laughter, babies, and our empty house already felt like a home.

Love,
Mom

Thursday, September 9, 2010

Dear Babies,

Since even my stretchiest tank top no longer covers my stomach, I must pull it down, down, all the way down so that the neckline practically scoops under my boobs, fully exposing my sports bra underneath. (Size 36 D from 34 barely B, *nice,* right?) Pair this classy look with skin-tight cropped maternity yoga pants and my ever-protruding belly button (hey, is that a belly button down your shirt or are you just excited to see me?).

This was what I looked like when I left the house this morning.

While out and about, I saw an advertisement nailed to a tree on 96th and Broadway: "Want to learn Hebrew and get help with math?"

I paused in front of the crumpled sign printed on neon orange paper, blinking at it from eye-level as if the dotted i in "with" would blink back at me. "Is it me, babies, or does this seem like a strange combo deal?" I said out loud.

Out loud because you're *here.*

I was so nervous trying to get pregnant. I was so nervous throughout the pregnancy. I'm so nervous thinking about you guys being born. (I am looking at a lifetime of worry, huh?)

I can't get down on my knees at church anymore but I still bow my head and squeeze my eyes shut so tight and say, "Please, God, *pleeeease,* we've come this far, please let everything be okay, please watch over us!"

You guys are people in here. How did this happen?

Frank Sinatra's "The Way You Look Tonight" came on while I was on hold with Pottery Barn scheduling a couch delivery.

"Some day, when I'm awfully low.
When the world is cold,
I will feel aglow just thinking of you,
And the way you look tonight."

I reached for your ten-week sonogram picture wedged in the hutch of my desk—the one where you look like you're in bunk beds—and I ran my thumbs over it. *"Yes you're lovely, with your smile so warm, and your cheeks so soft, there is nothing for me but to love you, and the way you look tonight."* I was the definition of getting choked up. I was literally choking on my tears. Diane from customer service clicked back and stopped herself mid-sentence to ask if I were all right.

I don't know if I'll ever be all right.

All I can do is sit here with my hand on my stomach, and feel the promise.

Love,
Mom

Monday, September 13, 2010

Dear Babies,

Big news today: The Starbucks Pumpkin Spice latte is back.

The fact that your father and I had our apartment packed up this morning and are moving out of New York City tomorrow could also be considered big news, but we're actually too busy to stop and process this life-changing event. Tomorrow we're moving to a place where everyone drives. Where people may or may not borrow sugar from one another. We're moving to Long Island. We're moving to *the suburbs.*

Knowing the movers would be here between 9:00 a.m. and 9:30 a.m. this morning, I told your dad to wake me up at 8:50 a.m. I was sure this would allow me ample time to physically maneuver getting out of bed, going to the bathroom, dressing, eating, and scanning the place for anything we would need to function in the barren apartment for the next 24 hours (i.e. clothing, toilet paper, a toothbrush, lemonade and a bag of roasted pumpkin seeds). Right.

At 9:02 a.m. the movers showed up.

Who says they'll be someplace between 9:00 a.m. and 9:30 a.m. and then shows up at practically nine on the dot? I had only washed and dressed and was one bite into my overstuffed egg salad sandwich when seven giant Russian men invaded the living room like gas-masked Nasa astronauts set to quarantine the San Fernando Valley in *E.T.* We were given specific orders: Anything NOT marked with an "x" would be boxed up and packed. By the looks of these guys, I knew this included me. I quickly took my sandwich, left, and ate it while sitting next to your father on a bench in the middle of Broadway. We sat looking forward and not talking, like two old people. I was thinking, "Should I pick up this glob of egg salad that just fell on the ground?" I don't know what your dad was thinking, but he looked like he could cry.

. . . Our apartment is now officially empty, except for our bed which we'll sleep on tonight, and an old couch that won't fit through the door. Your father is very upset about the couch. He wanted it as part of his master plan for the basement, which he thinks will be man-cave (which will become a playroom). I am not so secretly rejoicing about it. The couch is gross, babies, trust me. It was left here from the previous owners for this same reason. (And how many previous owners before that? Who owns this thing? And why have I been okay about it this whole time??) We have a house. We don't have to live with other people's smelly asses on our couch anymore. I only want to live with our smelly asses.

{Pause.}

You know what I mean.

Here I am, though, on the controversial couch for one last time, remembering how excited your father and I were when we bought this place three years ago. We'd been out all day at a christening in the Upper East Side, which turned into bar hopping on Second Avenue, which turned into convincing friends to come back to "our place" to order pizza even though it was completely empty except for the eternal couch. We sat on it surrounded by painters' canvases and step ladders, not minding the fumes, drinking wine from plastic cups and sharing a cheese pie.

Cheers, to the possibilities! we toasted as a young couple with the world in front of them.

And outside on the streets below us city lights flickered. The traffic, like a heartbeat, ebbed and flowed. . .

That's the beauty of a life that's alive. You can never imagine what the possibilities will be.

See you in our new home.

Love,
Mom

Tuesday, September 14, 2010

Dear Babies,

Andy Warhol has this mind-bending quote about how people think that what happens in movies is not real but actually it's life that is unreal: "The movies make emotions look so strong and real, whereas when things really do happen to you, it's like watching television—you don't feel anything."

I thought of this today on this bright, sunny Tuesday as your father and I drove over the Throgs Neck Bridge with our loaded car headed eastbound for Long Island, the sweeping New York City skyline glistening to our right and growing smaller and smaller as we drove leaving it behind. As a little girl coming over that bridge, all I ever wanted was to be a part of that skyline. I couldn't wait to move there after college. I was going to be Carrie Bradshaw, a writer, single in the city. Cue Carly Simon, *let the river run. . .* I met your father a month before I moved in, and we've been together ever since. I was never single in the city. With my dirty boat shoes, I am hardly Carrie Bradshaw. I colored a life there so different than anything that wide-eyed girl could have ever imagined. A crazy life. A small life. (I looked up a lot.) A life that was my own. As quickly as I jumped into the relentless current of New York City, today, I swim off.

I had envisioned this moment of change so differently. I pictured your father and I crying. Embracing. Lingering in an empty apartment as we removed the last picture frame from the mantel, turning around for one last look. . .

(Okay fine, we didn't have a mantel, that's the ending scene of the series finale of *Growing Pains*, but whatever.)

As we drove, I thought maybe Frank Sinatra's "New York, New York" would be on.

Meanwhile, I was on my phone with Nanny trying to give her directions to the house. She kept interrupting, listing all the food she was bringing. "There's eggplant, ziti, mashed potatoes, I made meatbawls for Mike. . ."

Your father was holding his phone an inch from his mouth shouting so the movers on speaker could hear him. "HELL-LOW?"

I don't even know what song was on, if there was even a song on at all. . .

People say man plans and God laughs.

He laughs, and bids us the ability to get through these life changing moments without breaking down hysterically like a scorned Susan Lucci character. Mr. Warhol was right: Life is not this hyper-charged soap opera. Stuff will happen, and you will go numb.

One minute you find yourself spinning in a circle underneath the throbbing strobe light with your arms thrown around someone's shoulders: "Oh my God! I'm at my senior prom!"

You hear your name called up to the podium: "Wow, I'm graduating *college*."

You're introduced to a room full of cheering family and friends, "For the first time, Mr. & Mrs. Denby!": "I'm *married*. This is my *wedding*. . ."

I was 22 when I met your father. We were kids, running around this city. And now. . . Now, I am propped up on fourteen pillows in a bed in a house in the 'burbs. I am rubbing my pregnant belly and feeling you guys kick. If I stick my neck out to the side, I can just about see my toes. Your

Supah Geek father is downstairs setting up one of our seven televisions.

And tomorrow is another day.

Love,
Mom

FOUR NAVEL ORANGES.

(THAT'S EIGHT ORANGES)

(THAT'S A LOT OF ORANGES)

Wednesday, September 15, 2010

Dear Babies,

Thirty-one weeks today and our doctor told me I was humongous. Not big. Not, "Wow, you've grown since your last visit!" Humongous, a word used by four-year-olds to describe elephants.

Under normal circumstances this might be cause for concern, but we were all celebrating, your father, grandparents, aunts and I. You guys are four and a half pounds each! I hear all of these stories about twins born prematurely, and you're such a good weight, already. *How blessed.* I'm currently carrying the equivalent of nine pounds of baby, but still, we're all healthy, everything is good.

Your cribs arrived today. Seeing how smushed you guys are in here on the ultrasound, your two little heads side by side, you should be very excited. Your new beds are definitely an upgrade.

I lingered in your room tonight, running my hands over the new, smooth mahogany. I tried to reach down and touch the mattresses but I got stuck on the railing. (Sorry.)

"Come to bed, babe," your father beckoned, coming up behind me cupping his palm on my shoulder.

I turned to take one last look after he flicked off the light.

Love,
Mom

Thursday, September 16, 2010

Dear Babies,

I saw some actress on *Access Hollywood* today talking about how Ashton Kutcher was her "pregnancy boyfriend," meaning she had dreams about him her whole nine months.

Please don't laugh, babies, but ours is Bradley Cooper.

Not much happens in the dreams. Often I'm checking into some hotel in Las Vegas, and he is up at the counter too, and then we start making small talk and he tells me he is in town shooting *The Hangover 2*. Sometimes he buys me a drink by the pool.

There's also this thing called your "celebrity baby," which is the famous person due to give birth around your same time. Ours are an eclectic crew: John Travolta and Kelly Preston, Celine Dion and her French husband, and Neil Patrick Harris and his partner. Two "older" couples and a gay man. Celine and Neil are even having twins! How very Hollywood of us.

Speaking of "Hollywood:" I have turned into the Sarah Connors of suburbia. Whereas two days ago I was still my old bug-saving self, carefully carrying a venomous tarantula in between two plastic cups out to safety, so far today I have killed a moth, multiple wasps, a spider that was so big it felt like I was killing a rabbit, and a mosquito with my bare hands. I lived with water bugs that looked like dinosaurs in my basement apartment on Thompson Street, but now, a gnat in my new home where my babies will live? *Take no prisoners.*

Love,
Mom

Monday, September 20, 2010

Dear Babies,

I was mindlessly washing my hands in the sink this morning, looking at my pale reflection in the bathroom mirror trying to ignore the fact that I look like Gollum from *Lord of the Rings* (I mean, did you notice that?) when it drifted into my mind: *The B. Cafe. . .*

The B. Café is a small restaurant by our apartment we just moved from in the Upper West Side.

It's okay.

It has outdoor seating.

It has really good French fries and mussels, if you're into that sort of thing.

But suddenly I was terribly missing The B. Café, so much I could've cried.

It's not that I miss the restaurant, babies. It's not that I even miss the city.

The restaurant was part of your father's and my repertoire. Like maybe we'd say, *what do you want do for dinner? Grab something out? B. Café?* And then we'd go—we'd know we could get a table—and he'd get a croque monsieur and I'd get a grilled Portobello on brioche.

(We sound a tad fancy, don't we?)

(Did you notice how I said "tad?")

I miss feeling settled in our life. Being in a routine. Not having to sit for an hour and untangle a ball of necklaces that became knotted in the move because "I won't have time to do it once the babies come." People love to tell me all the things I'm *never* going to do again. Sleep is a big one. Go to the gym. Get a manicure. This may be true but come on, won't I adjust? What, am I not going to write? (Can you feel the fear?)

You never went to the gym anyway, I want to say to these people. *Look at my pirate nails, do you think that I care?* When I'm a new mom and meet pregnant women, remind me not to say such things. I hope I say, *you will make time for the things you want to do.*

Some days I have to be home from nine to eleven to wait for the electrician. The cable guy. Direct TV. And then I flush a toilet and learn that it leaks. I pull down a shade so I don't terrify the neighborhood when changing and it comes crashing down.

Oh, I can't wait to be settled...

But as soon as we do get the house ready, you guys will be here. Life as we knew it and any sense of normalcy is *gone.*

I'm not so much scared, it's all just so surreal and hurts my head to think about, like the first time I saw *The Matrix* and that little kid kept saying, "There is no spoon."

Eh, what are we gonna do?

I'm sitting here with no pants on watching *Dancing with the Stars.*

Tomorrow I'll continue to complain to you guys about how full I am. Eating is tough again like it was in the beginning, only now I'm not hungry and don't want to eat anything (except soft pretzels dipped in Nutella). I'll muse about dumb things, like how embarrassed I am for celebrities in perfume commercials (they all whisper). The next day, maybe I'll tackle that pile of foreign objects in the basement also known as baby gifts from our shower this past weekend...

Just wait.

That's another thing people love to tell me. Just wait till that black poop comes in. Just wait till they get they start teething. Just wait till they start walking.

Well here I am, waiting.

Love,
Mom

Tuesday, September 21, 2010

Dear Babies,

Here's to us kickin' a in suburbia this morning.
{High five.}
{High five.}

Despite a minor mishap with the power rear door, I figured out how to use the new car, or should I say, any car, having not driven one regularly in oh, about *eight years*. (For the record, I think the key should have a button that says "push twice to open," because what, you're just supposed to *know* how to work a *car*?)

We went to the pediatrician, to Bed, Bath & Beyond and to Whole Foods. *Wow*. It felt so *good* to be out driving around a neighborhood, with trees! On more than one occasion I caught myself smiling in the rearview mirror. The beautiful tudor homes. Coming around the bend on Plandome Road and catching a sparkling view of the water peppered with sailboats.

I am driving around Manhasset in an SUV. . . who am I?

I was friendly to strangers, too.

(Kind of.)

I smiled at women in the stores. I let a man carry my groceries.

Our pediatrician this morning said that the best advice he can give me is not to listen to anyone's advice. "There is no baby in the world that is going to be like yours," he rationalized, "so, just because one woman uses a product and her baby breaks out in a rash doesn't mean yours will."

In other words, there is no right way to be a mom. . .

Oh I like him.

I'm tired tonight. Swollen. There is still so much to do. Loose wires are everywhere and those damn dust bunnies seem to have multiplied (as bunnies do), but I have less anxiety about it.

I think we're going to be okay.

I can't wait to buy us a pumpkin.

Love,
Mom

JICAMA.

Wednesday, September 22, 2010

Dear Babies,

This is what happens when you watch shows like *Desperate Housewives.*

You think that the insurance walkthrough guy at the door might actually be thinking *something* (wink, wink) as you answer out of breath and Sade's "No Ordinary Love" is faintly playing through the air. (After days of listening to the Hall & Oates station on Pandora, I decided to mix it up with Sting. The result was easy listening.)

I blushed thinking what this guy could be thinking.

Meanwhile, I am a moose—and I saw a moose on the Today Show this morning for getting an antler stuck on some family's swing set in Idaho, so I would know.

The only thing he could've been thinking was "wow, she's really sweating," not grossed out but concerned for my well-being.

At thirty-two weeks pregnant, I have ballooned. I am so swollen I have become an anomaly. People stop me on the street to ask if they can get me something, water, a chair.

It's dark out now and I am looking out the window.

There's a light on in the house across the street but I can't see any people.

I don't know any people.

Not one car has gone by.

(It sure is quiet out here in the 'burbs. . .)

When I was 23 and moved into the City, Poppy told me to look up. He said, "City people always look forward. Remember to look up at the sky. . ."

I'm looking up at the sky now. I can't recall the last time I saw so many stars. . .

I'm thinking of Poppy. I'm thinking of you. I'm thinking of your father. Tonight is his first night commuting home from the city after a work function. I wonder what time he'll get home. How he'll get home. Will he take a car. The train. He walked to the station this morning but now he can't walk back, it's starting to rain.

I soften my grip on the pulled back curtain and it swings in, closing the scene.

They say the whole world is a stage.

Doesn't that sound depressing? Like everyone is performing.

(Though careful, some people are.)

Maybe what they mean is that life is a series of curtains opening and closing, of scenes beginning and ending.

As I climb the stairs, brush my teeth, dim the lights, and another day fades to black.

Love,
Mom

Thursday, September 23, 2010

Dear Babies,

Today your Nanny and Aunt Krissy came over to help me organize our baby shower gifts.

They joked that I was going to write you a letter about how unhelpful they were, but aside from occasionally catching them sitting on the couch eating Doritos and watching *General Hospital*, they really were of great help.

(I tease them a lot. It's my role as the smart aleck in the family. But I'll let my guard down and tell you, and only you, how much I admire them, how they really are the best.)

So, you guys have twelve rubber ducks but no bottles or any of the 12,000 things I've been told we will "need." Looks like a trip to BuyBuyBaby is in order. I've become like a heat-seeking missile in that place. (A missile with coupons.) Organic stain remover? Back left corner. Toys? To the right. Bedding is upstairs. Okay going there is still a nightmare—but I like knowing I can get exactly what I need in every category at the same store. If only such places existed for all arenas of life. For instance, I need face wash, a wedding card and a big curbside garbage pail. . . Or did I just create Walmart?

Hmph.

Makes you appreciate the simplicity of an original idea. Filling a hole in the market, blah, blah, blah.

Love,
Mom

Friday, September 24, 2010

Dear Babies,

Grumpah brought Maga over for lunch today and to see the house. My mom went grocery shopping for us yesterday to prepare: One pound each of turkey, ham, genoa salami, provolone, bologna, American and Swiss cheese, a dozen rolls, and a box of Devil Dogs—for three people. One a barely functioning-about-to-burst pregnant vegetarian.

At age 83—her birthday is on Sunday—Maga was as beautiful and funny as ever. . .

Grumpah trimmed all of our hedges outside while we sat inside on the couch in the air conditioning listening to Frank Sinatra and talking about everyone else in the family. Coffee tawk with Sophia from *The Golden Girls* and Jabba the Hutt.

You know, growing up all I ever wanted was to be normal. For our family to be *normal.*

I'd go to friends' houses and see that nobody was yelling. Their dads weren't crouched in the bushes with the water hose, waiting to squirt unsuspecting friends—and *boyfriends*—at the door.

But here's a secret, babies: Nobody thinks their family is normal. Not even the normal ones. You'll save yourself some teenage angst if you accept this now.

You can't change people, so get over it, and eat a Devil Dog with your grandma.

Love,
Mom

Monday, September 27, 2010

Dear Babies,

I sat on the couch this morning in my black bathrobe and big fuzzy slippers like The Dude from *The Big Lebowski*, eating granola and watching Kathie Lee and Hoda, a sentence that will make future me green with envy.

We went to the post office to buy stamps for our baby-shower thank you notes, which Auntie Krissy was so nice to get for us and address but unfortunately did not take into consideration the cards' insane amount of glitter. (If people still send greeting cards, don't buy ones with glitter.)

There is a single square of green glitter on the tip of my nose I can see when I go cross-eyed, yet cannot get at to remove.

Where are all the automated machines? I huffed surveying the station. *You mean I have to wait on this line to talk to someone, just to buy stamps? What a waste of time. The Union Square station would never have stood for this!*

(I know, future self, punch away.)

"Do you have any of those automated stamp machines?" I asked the teller up at the counter. I was squinting, looking around, even behind him through to the next teller's window, in utter disbelief that thirty minutes from Manhattan a place could be *that* behind the times. *What, do you offer express mail, priority or pigeon?*

Once outside, when I couldn't get the car key to work—*is it one click or two, beep-beep, nothing, come on!*—I pretended this was intentional to the pack of high school students standing nearby, *because they cared*, and I walked to find a great French bakery everyone keeps asking if I'd tried. I knew it was around there *somewhere*. It started to rain, of course. I didn't have an umbrella, of course. A neon vested crossing-guard held up traffic for me—not schoolchildren—crossing Port Washington Boulevard. I felt the glares of a hundred SUV drivers upon me. All for a latte. And maybe a chocolate scone.

—Closed.—

When I got to the door I saw that the bakery is closed on Mondays.

I pressed my nose against the glass and peaked in the window taunted by militant rows of pastel macaroons.

. . . King Kullen was next on the agenda where I talked out loud to myself the whole time.

"Where is the cheese shop???" I grunted under my breath, annoyed when I couldn't find fresh unsalted mozzarella.

Yes, I called the dairy section of King Kullen "the cheese shop," as if we were in a seaside village with winding cobblestone streets, not a mega shopping center with a Payless, a GNC and a Rite Aid next door.

In the "daily fresh bakery" section, I squeezed all the baguettes listening for the right sound. "Hmph," I put each one down disappointed, not hearing the crunch I was looking for. "Too soft," I said like I was an expert when in actuality I had only learned to choose good bread this way from Jeanine Garofalo's character in the animated movie *Ratatouille* about a rat that can cook.

Don't even get me started about the lack of selection in the organic section.

—No vegan turkey salad? What the hell?!—

True, I was spoiled living in the Upper West Side among the city's best grocery stores—Zabar's, Fairway, Citarella. All the local markets, too, bakeries, and yes, even cheese shops.

But I think it's more than that.

Every time I leave the house I turn into Borat when he doesn't know how to work the elevator. He keeps going up, then down, up, then down. . .

Growing up Auntie Krissy and I loved the story of the Town Mouse and the Country Mouse. She was the Country Mouse, who preferred the safety of the simple life in the country. I, the Town Mouse, who risked the danger of the City for the chance of better food.

What if I'm starting to realize, what have I done?

What happens to the mouse who is excited to buy a nice house in the suburbs to raise her family in with a yard, and closets to hoard things in like giant packs of toilet paper and expired Ricola cough drops, then gets there and is like, *what have I done?*

—*Who moved your cheese? You did, dumbass!*—

What happens to her?

Love,
Mom

Tuesday, September 28, 2010

Dear Babies,

I met Nanny at BuyBuyBaby today to finish up shopping for you guys. Now I know why they call it "BuyBuy" Baby. I can spend at least $300 there in a heartbeat. On what?—*bombshell!*—I don't even know!

When we left and said good-bye to each other in the parking lot, she turned right to head back home and I turned left to head west. I felt sad for a moment. I wanted to go with her. I wanted to go back to the house I grew up in and sit on the couch and be taken care of. I wanted to have nothing to do for the rest of the afternoon but sit and watch TV.

Tired.

Oh, my feet.

I feel so full of baby.

But no.

I drove home—to our home—in the rain.

I unloaded the bags.

I made butternut squash soup.

While she will always be my mother and take care of me, now I am your mother and will take care of you. If I stopped to think about this I could freak myself out. Think that I'm not ready yet. That I am playing dress-up in a very expensive and slightly-spider-infested-in-the-basement dollhouse (I swear we are a holding set for a secret casting call for a new *Arachnophobia*).

One of the more annoying things people will tell you when they're trying to help is "don't think about it." *Genius! How'd you think of that?!*

They're right, though.

I'll try not to think about it.

I'll sit here and eat my soup.

Love,
Mom

PINEAPPLES.

Wednesday, September 29, 2010

Dear Babies,

Thirty-three weeks today, but as of our doctor's appointment this afternoon I am officially the size of a full-term forty week woman with a single baby.

{High-five.}

{High-five.}

Your father was nervous this morning. He took this haphazard pile of clothes for the hospital I've been stockpiling in the corner like a squirrel burying nuts—nursing bras, slippers, cheap pajamas, packs of giant cotton underwear that come in a pack of four—and dumped it into a shopping bag. He took it with him to work thinking he would meet me at our appointment, and we would not come home, at least without increasing our family by 200%.

But no, everything was good.

More of the same. We're big, but good.

I go back on October 13th for one more ultrasound and then, because Baby B is slightly transverse and there's a chance I could have a vaginal birth *and* a C-section, no thanks!, we're going to schedule a C-section for either October 25th or November 1st.

It feels weird to schedule your birthday like a hair appointment. I like to think that fate can still be a part of it. . .

The other day, the woman behind the counter of a local Mediterranean place told me she could read auras and that when I walked in the door she felt I had great energy. She said her boyfriend who had recently passed's birthday was on October 25th, and she was really feeling that day for your birthday, *without me saying a thing.*

We'll see if this is the new lunch deal: Fate and a falafel sandwich.

Love,
Mom

Thursday, September 30, 2010

Dear Babies,

We lost power today.

I was in the middle of doing laundry and washing pacifiers and figuring out what the hell to do with twelve rubber ducks of various sizes when I decided to break for lunch.

Cream of cauliflower soup.

I had to have it.

I cooked up my version of it, salivating, pausing occasionally to look out the window and wonder *where is this tropical storm Al Roker keeps talking about?* There was wind, but not a lot of rain. I was so happy when I reached the final stage of my preparation, the pureeing, and maybe adding a little more milk.

"What the?" I said as soon as I plugged in my handheld immersion blender (of all the things people will describe as the best thing ever, believe it or not this thing is it) and the electricity went out. I had flashbacks to 8:30 p.m. every Saturday night in college when all the girls on my sorority floor would blow dry their hair at the same time, and shuddered at the same fate for this house if you are two girls.

All the kitchen lights went out.

The fridge.

The stove.

"Hmm..."

I began to walk around the house flipping switches like the elephantine Columbo.

The dining room light.

The living room cable box.

The phones.

My computer.

I heaved up the stairs...

There, too, everything was off.

I called your father, whose immediate reaction was, "What d'ya do?," a suspicion I secretly harbored while thinking, *oh, crap, did my beloved immersion blender really cause the blackout?* And I said "blackout" dramatically, bitter after spending an entire season last year watching some show on ABC about what caused a mysterious worldwide blackout only for the damn thing to be canceled so now I'll never know. (See all the little ways life can torture you?)

I checked the circuit breaker in the garage with a flashlight like I actually knew what I was doing. Nothing.

I had to find out if it was just our house, or if the street was out. *If perhaps this blackout was worldwide, too.*

. . . A few years ago there was this guy at a Halloween party who dressed up as a tornado. He wore a black t-shirt and black pants, and hung plastic farm animals and Lego people from himself with about an inch of clear string so that when he spun, they would whirl around him.

I mention this now because as I headed off down our block, on which I still know zero people (welcome basket of muffins, where are you??), I was dressed as his tornado. A black t-shirt barely stretched over my belly. Black cropped yoga pants, barely pulled up over my behind. Stuck to me were flecks of cauliflower florets and yellow duck fuzz from when I was upstairs earlier putting away your new hooded critter towels.

(Okay, you caught me. I was actually trying them all on. I sat with the duck towel on for a bit, draped over my shoulders and the beak hood capped over my forehead like a really ridiculous Rocky.)

"Hello? Hello?!" I called with desperation like I had just been stranded in the woods for days without food or water to the few men surrounding a white van that read "1-800-Mr. Faucet" in a neighbor's driveway. I was waddling and panting, swinging my arms back and forth to pull me along. *Heave-ho!*

I am not being paranoid when I say the men began to laugh.

I would've laughed, too, if I were in their situation. Laughed, or cowered in a corner secretly dialing 311 to report an approaching and possibly rabid bear.

Turns out the neighborhood did lose power. Apparently I do live in the woods. Maybe there really are bears.

Three hours later when everything came back on, a repetitive "beeping" sound began to emit from the stove.

Beep. . . beep. . . beep. . .beep. . .

I didn't know what was causing it; I couldn't get it to stop. I cursed the thing.

I visualized taking an ax and hacking it to pieces.

I empathized with Jack Nicholson's housebound character in *The Shining.—Here's Johnny!—*

An hour went by like this until I noticed the wrong time on the stove's digital clock was flashing in sync with the beeping. *Could it be?* I set the right time and voile, the problem was solved.

The British have an expression Keep Calm and Carry On.

How about Keep Calm and *Think*.

Think, babies, *think*.

Love,
Mom

Friday, October 1, 2010

Dear Babies,

I don't want to rush you in any way, but, I have to tell you, I was putting away (*cough*, playing with) some of your toys earlier and this Captain Calamari Pirate thing is awesome. He has an eye patch, and one of his tentacles is a squishy hook. . .

Love,
Mom

Monday, October 4, 2010

Dear Babies,

Look, it's no big deal.

I wouldn't even say anything to you guys if society didn't have such an obsession with them, but, I was taking your new bottles out of their boxes today and noticed that they all say "BreastFlow."

I know, it's so stupid.

What are we, five? Or in your case, in utero? Snickering over boobs and underwear?

I've been obsessing over bottles. I've bought about fourteen different kinds. *What's the best??*, I ask everyone. Apparently Dr. Brown is no good for me: *With twins? You'll hate cleaning all of those parts.* I hear Born Free a lot. Avent. A stern Jamaican baby nurse swore by Playtex Drop-Ins. "But I'd be throwing out a plastic bag every single time they eat?" I dared to question in a voice that made Alvin and the Chipmunks tenors by comparison. "Isn't that, like, really bad for the environment?" She gave me a look, and sometimes looks can say way more than words.

These "BreastFlow" ones come recommended to avoid, wait for it, nipple confusion. Yes, apparently by planning on breast *and* bottle feeding you guys I will be messing you up right out of the gate. *Now I'll never be Mother of the Year!* People say the two hot-button topics you never bring up at a party are politics and religion. But my gosh, parenting could cause the next world war. Breast milk versus formula. Glass bottles versus plastic. When do you stop breast feeding. *Ah, there goes the Mother of the Year, accepting her award with a five-year-old attached to her boob, you can't see him under the podium...*

I'm a planner. What if I can't make enough milk for you guys, or any at all? Won't I need a backup plan? Will I really be less of a mother for giving you, horrors, *formula*? Come on. I can think of a million other ways I can screw you up besides that.

Relax, I'm kidding. Remember you are *humans*, which means you'll be perfectly screwed up all your own, and I mean that in the best possible way.

Love,
Mom

CANTALOUPES.

Wednesday, October 6, 2010

Dear Babies,

Thirty-four weeks today and I just don't feel well.

I'm sorry, I don't mean to complain.

I know you guys have it tight in there and are probably pretty uncomfortable yourselves. Baby A, I picture you saying to Baby B, or maybe vice versa, "Oh, you're still here?," like an old married couple at the diner.

My feet are so swollen, you guys.

I'm so. . . bone. . . tired. I feel as if I can barely hold up my head.

My breaths are slow and heavy like Darth Vader's.

This alien stomach housing you just shoots out and out, and walking is like steering a ship. I have to literally pick up my belly when I sit to keep it from sagging on the chair, because yes, the only way I can sit is with my legs spread wide open to make room for this egg, which means *yes*, I have to lift up my belly like a sack of potatoes to pee.

Forget lying down. Forget sleeping.

Baby A, you constantly have the hiccups. Baby B, what is the fascination with my ribs?

I now have carpal tunnel syndrome in both wrists, not from writing, *please*. The closest I've come to anything literary is this Shakespeare mug I'm currently using, and I'm not even drinking from it, rather dipping a bagel into my tea which is kind of gross, but kind of really amazing. Apparently all the swelling is pressing down on my nerves. I picked up a plate before and shrieked in pain nearly dropping it on the ground. I hope this goes away when you're born. Otherwise, how will I carry you?

Still, *I am not complaining...*

Take me out of the equation and everything is fine. Everything is good.

I bought us a "real" ironing board yesterday, one of those big ones a 50's housewife stood behind in an apron. That's actually why I did not write to you. After carrying it, along with other necessities from Home Goods including a giant sign that says "Eat, drink and be merry," my back was in so much pain that I was bent parallel to the floor.

—"Time has fallen asleep in the afternoon sunshine."—

That's one of my favorite quotes. It's the line from *Fahrenheit 451* that Guy Montag reads accidentally and sparks his interest in the forbidden books he's been burning.

Let's go find a quiet spot on a couch somewhere in the sun. Close our eyes and try to sleep, like a cat.

Love,
Mom

Thursday, October 7, 2010

Dear Babies,

I'm becoming grouchy now, like an old irritable person who doesn't feel well and doesn't want to be taken care of, but needs to be.

(Good luck taking away my keys.)

I officially have zero tolerance for annoying people and things, both of which are found in the commercial for that new movie *Life As We Know It* starring Katherine Heigl and Josh Duhamel.

This is the movie's premise on IMDB.com:

Two single adults become caregivers of an orphaned girl when their mutual best friends die in an accident.

I mean, come on???!!!

Even the song from the trailer is torturous, "Hey, Soul Sister" by Train. If I were able to hoist myself up from the ten pillows I'm propped up on in a timely manner I swear I would chuck one at the TV screen.

But no.

I am slow. . .

I am now sporting ace bandages on each wrist. . .

I am dependent on others to help me get up, which is apparently every seven minutes to pee. . .

I am a prisoner with the song "Hey, Soul Sister" on repeat in my head. I would do anything to make it stop. . .

Forget water boarding. I must tell Dick Cheney about this.

Love,
Mom

Friday, October 8, 2010

Dear Babies,

Today started off so respectable. I sat at the kitchen island and read a newspaper. I got my morning news from CNN instead of Kathie Lee and Hoda.

Then, I decided that it *might* be abnormal that the itching I had last night was so bad that I had to spend the three a.m. hour in a bathtub with my hands in wine chiller sleeves and my feet immersed in ice, so I looked it up online. Within seconds I diagnosed myself with a fatal liver and gallbladder disease. My body was filling up with bile salts by the minute that would lead to stillbirth.

—*Oh, my God!*—

Immediately I hopped off my stool and called our doctor, whose number I've upgraded to the "Favorites" list on my phone.

"Hi, Maureen!" I said when I got the nurse, like we're old chums. It's hard to imagine a time when I didn't say our doctor's name on a daily basis. It's hard to imagine a time when I won't. When I'll revert back to yearly visits, like everyone else. *Wah.*

"If you had a life-threatening liver disease brought on by increased pregnancy hormones in the third trimester, you would have *severe* itching. . . all over. It would be ferocious," she said.

I paused, trying to decide if my itching was indeed ferocious. *Ferocious, like a lion?* "Umm, I mean," I psychosomatically began scratching my wrists, "it's irritating, but. . ."

I envisioned said lion, and concentrated on where exactly on my body did it itch. *ROAR.* Nowhere, I concluded, *but what if I'm wrong?*

"I *did* scratch under my armpit last night," I actually said to a medical professional. "And my neck, it was kind of red when I woke up. I could've been scratching that, too."

This woman is not only a miracle worker who brings babies into this world but a patient saint.

She assured me my case did not present itself as "ferocious."

She told me to watch it.

To call her if it intensifies and come in for a blood test. Otherwise, I will see her on Wednesday and we can do blood work then.

I hung up and gazed out the window.

Grumpah was over, cutting down dead branches in our swamp of a backyard. He must have gashed the tip of his nose on something and was standing on the patio with a snowball of bloody paper towels pressed to his face. He caught eye contact with me and waved, like this was all standard, just another Friday. And I scratched my forearms, my scalp, my chin. . .

Love,
Mom

Tuesday, October 12, 2010

Dear Babies,

I have a sinus infection.

I mean on top of everything—the itching! the skin stretching! the heartburn! the alien stomach with visible lumps of elbows, feet and heads! carpal tunnel in both wrists! the loss of walking, breath and sleep!—now I'm so congested my eyes and nose are oozing green puss and oh the pressure behind my forehead and ears.

Come on!

Worse, I feel guilty about it.

I am sorry I am sick right now.

I am sorry I can't be strong for you. That all I can do is lay here belly up like a seal on the beach. I didn't write to you yesterday because I actually followed doctor's orders and rested. Okay, not by choice, Aunt Krissy kidnapped me and took me out to Nanny's because no one trusted that I would actually relax, but once I was there, I was good. Nanny walked in with a shopping bag from Panera Bread—she'd bought one of every soup on the menu. I watched television and read three magazines, and I felt like an eighty-year-old for not knowing who half the people in *People* were, especially the musicians.

If your father's and my nightly complaint that "nothing is on" has given you the impression that primetime television is bad, you'd be horrified by daytime. At one point this afternoon my best option was a show on Animal Planet called *Animal Cops, San Francisco*, as opposed to the other franchises of the show, *Animal Cops, Detroit* and *Animal Cops, Houston*. Yes, babies, this is real. I mean, how different can the animal cops be from city to city? *Animal Cops, Supai, Arizona.*

Nanny reminded me that I was born with a sinus infection.

She said my eyes were crusted shut and I was a "huge, pink, completely bald oozing ham." (Memories!)

Maybe there's poetry, then, in the fact that I might be bringing my babies into the world the same way.

We'll find out tomorrow. Based on tomorrow's ultrasound we're scheduling your birthday.

Love,
Mom

HONEYDEW MELONS.

Wednesday, October 13, 2010

Dear Babies,

The good news is I get to wear my Halloween costume of Peter Griffin from *Family Guy*.

The bad news is that my train wreck of a body needs to carry on like this for another two and a half weeks.

You had to hear what an idiot I sounded like today with the doctor (oh, you probably did), stating my case on why we should schedule our C-section for earlier. *I'm so tired but I haven't slept in days because of the itching, I'm in my own personal* Nightmare on Elm Street. *I can barely do that thing, what's that thing,* breath. At thirty-five weeks, you guys are the size of two honeydew melons, a little over five pounds each. Sure, it's uncomfortable. (Two *melons*, the feeling of having a bowling ball shoved down my chest and one shoved up where the sun don't shine.) But then I thought of a *Family Guy* episode where they take stab at Julia Roberts and show her red-maned head and big toothy smile growing bigger and bigger until it ultimately explodes while she boasts, "Me, ME, it's all about MEEEEEEEEEEEEE!" Well, that was me. Simply put, the longer you guys stay in here, the better off you are. Our doctor says everything is "great." So take me out of the equation. Sleeping is overrated. I have the rest of my life to breath. I get to hold you soon, so everything truly is great.

November 1st, babies.

8:45 a.m.

See you there.

Love,
Mom

Thursday, October 14, 2010

Dear Babies,

Nanny came over today to help with things, do the laundry, unload the dishwasher, offer me ten thousand things to eat.

"Do you remember what we were doing last year on November 1st?" I asked her while breaking from our chores over a nice little afternoon snack she threw together: Bread, olives, rice balls, slices of salami and provolone rolled into scrolls on a plate—for the two of us. "You guys were in the city for the Marathon. . . "

Last year, on your pending birthday, Grumpah was attempting to beat his previous year's record in the New York City Marathon. Marathon Sunday is one of the greatest days in New York City, if you ask me. The crisp fall weather. Everyone out on the streets. He had run a three-twenty-something in 2008, and in 2009 was looking to break it with three-twenty-something-less. (He did. When he runs he is not too far behind the men from Zimbabwe. I hope you guys are athletic like him. If not athletic then at least as equally dedicated and determined.)

"You guys came in and stayed over on Halloween, remember?" I reminisced. "We went out to dinner. . ." I looked in her eyes and knew what she was thinking, and knew I had to acknowledge it, too. "Mickey stayed at my apartment." As in Mickey, our dog who died this past August. "He was up all night, huffing and puffing, eyeing the couch and not wanting to sleep on the floor, poor spoiled thing. It was before we knew he was sick."

Her eyes swelled with water.

"We went to the Italian restaurant that was so good," she said after a few seconds, blinking back the tears. "I had the lasagna. Next time, I'll get the scallops."

Meanwhile, I blinked back tears of my own. A lot of things about that weekend were before.

Friends who had gotten pregnant through fertility treatments told us we would forget about everything, all the "bad stuff," once we got pregnant. You do, in some ways, but you also don't.

Last year on Marathon Sunday your father and I had just completed our third fertility treatment and were awaiting the results to see if we were pregnant. Things had not gone well. We did not have our hopes up. It is one thing for "Little Bit o' Luck" from New York Lotto to tell you, "hey, you never know." It is another for a white-coated doctor after a month of painful daily injections that did not come cheap.

That morning, while eating H&H bagels at my kitchen table with songs like Europe's "The Final Countdown" and Jay-Z's "Empire State of Mind" playing over NBC's broadcast of the race, I got an email from a friend telling me she was "preggo." (Her word, not mine.) Oh, the stabbing pain in my heart when I read those words. I was happy for her, don't get me wrong, it's just. . . one of the hardest parts of having trouble getting pregnant is that you feel like everyone around you is, and effortlessly so.

(People aren't mind readers, babies. Sometimes we expect them to be.)

Very few people knew what I was going through. And those who did, did not know how to treat me—especially friends who apparently sneezed and got pregnant, four times.

I would end up smiling to people to make them feel better, saying "it's okay, just treat me normal!," when I was grasping for normal in my own skin. I knew I was supposed to relax—"the minute I stopped thinking about it, I got pregnant!" chirped everyone, *gee, thanks for the tip!*—when during treatments you can't exercise, do yoga, drink alcohol, take a hot bath, any of the things that might help you to. It's so hard to stay positive. It's so hard not to become someone you don't recognize. It's so hard to be in that cycle of hope, loss, and heal. . .

I did not think I was pregnant. Still, to be cautious, I only had a few glasses of wine at the Marathon party that day—a rarity for Marathon Sunday where bloody Mary's at the bars along First Avenue notoriously flow all day into night.

I felt like a fool. Like I was pretending to be pregnant when I knew in my heart that the chances of that being true were very, very slim. I sat in a windowsill at the New York Athletic Club perched above the endless stream of runners snaking across Central Park South, nursing a pinot grigio and pitying myself like a bad drunk.

If Little Bit o' Luck had told me on that day that exactly one year later I would be in a hospital delivering two healthy twin babies, I would never have believed him.

While dwelling on the past can be dangerous, it is important to look back sometimes to see how far you've come and how much you've learned. How strong you've become. Life is so amazingly unpredictable, babies. You never know what the next moment will bring.

Or should I say, hey, you never know.

Love,
Mom

Friday, October 15, 2010

Dear Babies,

Grumpah brought Maga over again.

They arrived at the door at 10:30 a.m. with a dozen bagels, two pounds of cream cheese and a box of Dunkin Donuts and set it all out on my kitchen island in a spread that rivaled the brunch from Sandi Shulman's bat mitzvah in 7th grade.

I knew then that it was going to be one of those days.

I forced down my bagel, hungry but full at the same time.

Maga started pushing me to have a donut.

I did not want one.

I physically could not stomach one.

I haven't had a donut for breakfast since the Smurfs were on and I didn't think it was weird that they were turquoise, topless and that their pants were connected to their shoes.

I already had heartburn and was so, so full.

"HAVE ONE!" she ordered, not taking no for an answer.

"Okay, thanks!" I sang nervously as I chose a sizable donut with chocolate icing and colored sprinkles.

As much as I wanted to vomit, I'm not gonna lie, it was delicious.

Upon finishing, Grumpah, a typical Italian male, rose from his chair and took a seat on the couch leaving the clean-up for the women, even though "the women" were his eighty-year-old mother and daughter pregnant with twins. *(Role model!)* While cleaning up, I watched Maga pick out an onion bagel and hide it away under a napkin on a counter to the side.

"This will be my lunch, for lay-tuh," she whispered.

"Okay, but you don't have to hide it, no one will take it," I whispered back.

She ignored me and began making neat little piles of all the crumbs.

. . . So there we were sitting on the couch with me in the middle, snug as three bugs in a teeny rug, except apparently I was the only one who was actually snug. They were freezing. My dad kept his hands in his zip-up's pockets. My grandma didn't take off her coat.

"I bet if you made a fi-yuh the whole room would warm up," she suggested not so subtly.

I was in capri leggings and a v-neck t-shirt.

"I bet," I replied, making it clear that, yes, I was aware of the heating effects of fire but was not about to make one. The thermostat read 68 degrees. "I'm sorry, you guys, I haven't been cold since March. I have no concept of temperature, are you cold?"

"No!" the two beanpoles lied, shivering as they turned blue.

In charge of the remote control, Grumpah chose a nice, light, fluffy family movie for us to watch on a dreary Friday afternoon: Russell Crowe in *A Beautiful Mind*.

My grandma had never seen it before, so my dad explained every scene to her—"See that guy? He's not real"—which prompted her to recount all the people she knew from the senior center who had Alzheimer's, were dying from Alzheimer's, or had recently died from anything. *Ira?* Dead. *It was his liv-uh.* And this was all done in the dark, for after being accused of keeping every light in the house on and running my electricity bill "through the roof"—"What's the matta? You got every light on!" *"Um, well, no, I don't have every light on. I have this light on, because we're in this room"*—I didn't want to hear it anymore, so I turned off that one light.

   All the while telling me to relax. . .
   All the while telling me to put my feet up. . .
   All the while telling me to have another donut. . .

Love,
Mom

Tuesday, October 19, 2010

Dear Babies,

Remember our walks around the reservoir in Central Park?

Remember the turtles?

Remember listening to Van Morrison? Or Bob Marley once it got warm? Remember the time I cried like a crazy person when "Baby Mine" from the *Beaches* soundtrack came on?

Remember when we were so sick we couldn't eat anything without feeling like we just did tequila shots on spring break in Cancun?

Remember eating croutons and ranch...

Drinking nothing but chocolate milk...

And then there were the better days when we felt good and strong and *hungry.* When we ate all those eggs. When we wore shoes that could tie and took advanced exercise classes at Physique 57. Sometimes on the way home we'd pick up dinner, falafel pitas or Chinese food. Shrimp fried rice. Broccoli in brown sauce and we would have to specify "brown sauce" because the garlic sauce made us sick. *Remember?*

Everyone said this would happen, just as people say you will look back on pictures and see that you were never as fat, brace-faced, whatever as you thought you were. (This, babies, is true—except for in college when you might be bloated from drinking beer five nights a week and be inspired to try a pixie cut like a late-nineties Gwyneth Paltrow when oh yeah, you don't look anything like Gwyneth Paltrow, and you may actually look worse.) But for someone who generally did not "enjoy" pregnancy—I hated feeling sick, limited, and was a nervous wreck the whole time—here I am already starting to miss it. My swollen feet are becoming a distant memory. Despite all the ailments I'm experiencing right now, I am going to *miss* having you guys in here. I will miss having you with me all the time. I will pass a pregnant woman on the street and feel that pang in my heart again, not because I long to feel what she feels, but now because I *know* what she feels.

People smile in photographs for a reason. We are all wonderful editors collecting moments to look back on and say see, everything *was* great. The past is always a simpler time because it is behind you, and that means you already survived. Trust me, your first love was not that pretty or cute, but as we grow older, they become dynamite. Life grows fonder in memory.

It is with these sentiments that I recall one warm, sunny day my senior year of college. I was driving to class in my friend's red convertible Chrysler LeBaron, a cool car at the time. My hair was blonde and in pig tails (hold comments) and I had these aviator sunglasses on. "You guys," she said, stopping at a red light and turning down the radio as U2 belted *It's a beautiful day*, "we have it really good." With each passing day bringing us closer to graduation, we knew the freedom of nightly parties and the days of cruising around together were numbered. We knew we had to savor this time, and yet, *how*?

Thirty-six weeks pregnant, I wish I had the answer.

Love,
Mom

CRENSHAW MELONS.

Thursday, October 21, 2010

Dear Babies,

I was too exhausted to write last night.

Exhausted after our doctor's appointment, which went well again. It's too crowded in here to get actual measurements on you guys, but you are now the size of Crenshaw melons.

I was exhausted after getting jerked around in the backseat of Grumpah's car as he drove me home from the City after our appointment. He had the Yankee game blasting through the static on AM radio. I kept trying to drink this stupid decaf coffee, basically scalding black water. Eventually he had to pull over so I could empty it on the side of the road in defeat.

I was exhausted after getting home and talking to Auntie Krissy and finding out that Maga was in hysterics when earlier no one had picked up her calls. Apparently she'd panicked and thought I had gone into labor, for that's what it means to be Italian, babies. There is no calm. There is no reasoning. An unanswered telephone means something is *wrong*.

When Auntie Krissy finally calmed her down and explained that everything was okay, that I was just at the doctor for a scheduled appointment and that everything was fine, she also mentioned that you guys are really big in size. Maga then proceeded to tell her how BIG my father had been as a baby. Now, I'd always heard that my father weighed maybe 7 lbs when he was born. There were never any stories there. But now that it's come out that you guys are "big" for twins, forget it. Last night Maga had Grumpah being born at mythic proportions. Huge. Call the Guinness

Book of World Records. She said he was so big that she had no fluid left and she had to do "uh dry birth." Because of this barren dessert that was my grandmother's birth canal my father was born with scales all over his body. He shed these a few weeks later "like uh snake," and then he finally grew normal skin. (*Italians also rewrite medical books.)

So, I was so exhausted, I went straight to bed.

I woke this morning after a night of twisting and turning, trying to maneuver getting up to pee every hour randomly on the :02's, with your father standing over me whispering, "Hey, do you feel anything?" *Do I feel anything? I am delirious. I am aching from my feet to my back to my plummeted ribs to my arm where I just got a flu shot. I am nervous that I'm going to have a contraction and not realize I'm in labor until it's too late. Where should I begin?* "Do you want me to take a later train? I feel bad leaving you alone."

But I smiled, or rather forced a smile. "Babe, I am far from alone."

People say that you are born alone and you die alone, but that is not true. When you are born I will be there, babies, whether it be in a hospital, in this bedroom or in the back of a cab. (Preferably the former, please.)

Don't worry. Forever, I will be there.

Love,
Mom

Friday, October 22, 2010

Dear Babies,

Day and night my thoughts are consumed by you.

(And Benihana. That smell emanating from the restaurant's manicured gardens is intoxicating. Just saying.)

"Get a life," you're probably saying, but the truth is I don't really have a life right now.

My life used to be living in the city and waking up around seven and eating breakfast while reading the Wall Street Journal and going to the gym and coming home and showering and then working at my desk all day in our one bedroom apartment until your father would come home. And every afternoon around three I would hear music from the lessons at the school across the street. "La Vie en Rose" on the trombone sounded good. The Mexican Hat Dance, not so much.

That was my life.

Now, obviously, all that is gone.

I don't mean "gone" in a dramatic, negative way. More like, a chapter has closed, and I'm waiting for the next one to begin. I know everything will change once you guys get here, so until then, I'm in this weird in-between stage. Where my body is no longer mine. Where I pause with every twitch and twinge and wonder *is this labor?* Where everyone calls me every five seconds to check in. So far, a record-breaking four calls from Nanny today.

It's not even 10:00 a.m.

Love,
Mom

Monday, October 25, 2010

Dear Babies,

The clock struck noon today and so far, nothing.

Twelve hours down, twelve more to go.

I feel like Ebineezer Scrooge waiting for the ghost of Christmas past, waiting for something to happen: *Today was the day that psychic had predicted you would be born, so, here we are. . . is that??. . . nope, still nothing.*

I did lose feeling in my right thigh. Now the whole leg is swollen as opposed to just from the knee down, which for consistency might be better?

My heartburn is so bad that I'm in this constant state of regurgitation.

My wrists kill, but I can't wear my braces anymore because the itching underneath them is just too maddening. And they sort of smell like cheese.

My lips are all chapped from drooling while sleeping, thanks to the night-guard I have to wear to help with the underbite I've developed. Apparently it's not uncommon for your whole mouth to change during pregnancy. It's—where's my favorite word, as with every other messed up thing that's happened to my body the past nine months—*"normal!"*

My belly button is not only sticking out like a turkey thermometer but is also really red and irritated and kind of bunky.

But, labor? No. Nothing yet.

Mimi came over before. When leaving she said in her lovely-as-always Texas accent, "All right, hon-ay, see you on Monday!"

Come on, babies, let's wait until our scheduled date on Monday. Don't come today. Let's sit here. Let's wash onesies. Let's scribble all the different combinations of your names on paper over and over again...

At least let me try to shave my legs and get a pedicure first. I am a beast.

Love,
Mom

Tuesday, October 26, 2010

Dear Babies,

It's just crazy how we are going to be thirty-seven weeks tomorrow.

How I ate a huge piece of pumpkin cake from Stop & Shop covered with fluorescent orange icing for dinner.

How I seriously could not figure out before that the incessant ticking following me everywhere was from my own watch. Tick, tick, tick, tick.

It's crazy to think how this time next week you guys will be here.

—*Tick, tick, tick, tick.*—

Time to take our weekly picture for our Baby Bump app. Your father keeps having to step farther and farther back to fit me in the frame.

Love,
Mom

STALKS OF SWISS CHARD.

Thursday, October 28, 2010

Dear Babies,

Emotions are running high.

Everyone is nervous, excited, even crying—except for me.

I am refilling the salt box.

Shredding old papers I've had sitting on my desk.

Manically washing all of your sheets, bibs, and blankets.

Making sure the ties on your bumper are tied tight, just so.

Practicing popping your car seats in and out of the double stroller.

Adjusting the tightness of your seat belt straps.

Stashing burp cloths and Purell pumps all around the house.

Babies, this is it.

But when will I feel like a mother? Like I know what I'm doing? Like you guys are two breathing human beings we *created* with minds, hearts, and personalities of your own?

Monday morning?

Next week?

Next year?

(College?)

How will I be me one day, and the next, be a cow able to produce milk? How does that kick in?

How will I know what you need when you're crying? I see these mothers with their babies at restaurants. The way they pick them up and handle their wobbly heads like pros. They dig through grossly overstuffed diaper bags and fish out the right antidote. A pacifier. A bottle. A tiny giraffe named Sophie. How do they know? *(Why can't they just tell me?)*

This time last year, to cheer me up, your father took me to see the Yankees win the World Series. It was freezing. His company gave him tickets and we sat in the very last row with the wind cutting us every which way. He bought me peanuts. I was bundled in a long white sweater and a black knit ski hat and shearling-lined winter gloves. A green wooly scarf coiled twice around my neck. A red-faced man heckled me, "oh come on, it's not *that* cold out." "I am a weenie," I had replied, as it started to snow and your dad pulled me in close. . .

Yesterday your dad was at Yankee Stadium for a work conference being urged by his coworkers to hurry home to his pregnant wife.

Life changes just like that.

{Snap.}

I hope as quickly I will snap into mom mode.

I hope. . .

I am scared. . .

(Though I'm really not a weenie.)

In the meantime, I'll stay busy to not think about it.

I have these hangars that divide your closets into sizes like in a store.

0-6 months. . .

3-6 months. . .

All the way up to two years.

How cool is that?

Love,
Mom

Friday, October 29, 2010

Dear Babies,

We did our pre-op blood work at the hospital today. We'll all set for Monday.

You started kicking when our favorite song came on in the car home, Bob Marley's "Three Little Birds." *Remember how much I played that the beginning of our pregnancy?* That was a lifetime ago. Everything that has happened since then, everything that has ever happened, it all gets lumped now into "before."

Before...

I remember when I was an editorial assistant at *More* I went to a seminar presented by the American Society of Magazine Editors on how to make it to the next step. *How to climb your way up the masthead,* or something like that. There were all of these top level editors there from popular magazines, and I believe it was someone from *Time Out New York* who said, "No one is going to save you. No one is going to come tap you on the back."

If you want something in life, babies, you have to go get it. Never get stuck. I implore you to work hard and never give up on your dreams and your goals.

I wanted to have a baby.

I never gave up.

A family at the pizza place tonight stopped me as I waddled by on my 20th trip to the bathroom. "Excuse me, I'm sorry," they said, "but we have to ask, how many babies are in there?"

"Two," I answered.

They'd bet each other three.

Tears welled up as I passed them.

"You okay?" your dad asked helping me slide back into the table.

I grinned the grin of triumph.

"Never better."

Love,
Mom

Saturday, October 30, 2010

Dear Babies,

We did it.

We made it to our long awaited manicure and pedicure today.

{High five.}

{High five.}

The best part is, it only cost $31! The same manicure, pedicure and Daniel-Day-Lewis-lip-wax at my old place on Broadway would've cost $60!

At home we're busy getting ready for you.

We're changing light bulbs.

Stocking toilet paper.

Re-filling antibacterial hand soaps.

Doing laundry.

We're trying to think of everything we can possibly take care of now so that when you guys finally arrive we can fully focus on you—whatever that means.

Your dad put on R.E.M. as a joke. "It's the end of the world as we know it, but I feel fine." Partly as a dig to me, knowing how much I loathe, despise, detest—keep going with words meaning "dislike" here—the band; partly to find the right song to convey what we were feeling. Then he put on a nursery rhyme version of Pearl Jam's "Better Man."

I promise: We will only play the real "Better Man" for you.

Some of the children's songs out there are more torturous than R.E.M.

One more day. . .

Love,
Mom

Sunday, October 31, 2010

Dear Babies,

Today has been a Halloween to remember, and not just because of the absence of alcohol (though, that probably helped).

Despite the ghosts, the goblins, the bad Wes Craven marathons, and the small fact that this time tomorrow your father and I will be the parents of two children, we are not scared.

We're anxious.

We're excited—so excited beyond words—to see you. To hold you. To take your tiny hands in ours. To finally find out, what *are* you? Who are you? We can't wait to give you names and to meet the two toothless, bald-headed angels who have already captured our hearts so much it hurts.

It hurts.

But strangely, we are not scared.

Tomorrow is All Saints Day, a solemn Catholic holiday commemorating all the saints.

I'm not a holy roller or anything, babies, but I do believe in faith. I believe that faith—in anything, not just God or religion but spirituality, energy, faith in the universe, in meaning, in something bigger out there than ourselves—helps to see us through.

When your father and I were trying to get pregnant, I prayed to so many saints asking for help.

I prayed to Saint Gerard, the Patron Saint of Mothers.

I got down on my knees and dropped my head into my hands at church—partly to mask that I was crying in public, partly from the weight of desperation—in front of the altar of Saint Anne, Mary's mother.

Saint Christopher.

Saint Anthony.

Saint Jude.

Saint Francis, and all of his animals.

Your dad's Aunt Rita in Texas lit so many candles to Our Lady of Guadalupe for us that her husband, Uncle Lee, was afraid she might burn down the house.

Nanny and Auntie Krissy lit candles in church every week, too.

Every morning throughout this pregnancy—and I mean it, every single morning since that blessed March 10th afternoon when we were sitting on the couch watching *The Blind Side* one minute and we got the phone call that we were pregnant the next—before I would step a club of a foot out of bed or even waddle to the bathroom, I have continued to pray to these saints. I'd thank them for you guys. I'd give *thanks* for this brand new day I had with you, knowing that each moment with you was a gift. I'd ask them to watch over you, to be with you, to keep you healthy and safe. . .

To throw in an extra dose of crazy, I also wished on every "eleven" that would turn on the clock. *5:11, 6:11, 7:11.* Now, technically this has no meaning and is not a known superstitious "thing." It was something I made up and started doing one morning as I ate an English muffin because the two single digits of "eleven" on the microwave reminded me of you. More times than I can count I wished on those ones, focusing on those two red lines, individuals together. I wished that we would have a safe and healthy pregnancy. That both of my babies would carry full term and be born big, strong and healthy. . .

Tomorrow is 11/1, All Saints Day, your birthday.
And for that, I say, thank you.
Happy Birthday, babies.
We did it.

I Love You,
Mom

THEY'RE HERE. . .

Wednesday, December 1, 2010

Dear Babies,

It's 7:00 a.m. and I am hooked up to a breast pump watching a strange yellow liquid expel from my body through giant purple nipples into a contraption that looks no more legitimate than the flux capacitor from *Back to the Future.*

It's hard to believe one month ago today I was strapped to a gurney—yes, strapped, by the pressure of six large men in scrubs—with my doctor reaching up and into what must have been my ribcage to pull out "the high one."

I don't know what I thought a C-section was, but clearly it was not that.

You feel things.

You hear things.

You are awake and see blood splattered on the other side of a blue hanging curtain and on the blaring florescent lights above like a crime scene from *Dexter.*

"I am a horse," I quipped to the army of scrubs surrounding me through clenched teeth, writhing in pain, in reference to the unfortunate fact that while my body from the hips down was numb from the spinal anesthesia, my torso was not. They were poking my ribs like a piece of meat—*"You feel that? You do?"*—surprised I was feeling more than I should. "It takes a lot to knock me out!" I added, a little too enthused.

To this one of the anesthesiologists, a small-eyed British man, unhinged the table I was lying on and sent me flipping upside down. "There is room for only one sarcastic wank-a," I imagined him saying underneath his blue paper mask. Instead he cried to the army, "HOLD OFF!" as my arms were outstretched on either side of me horizontally and my numb feet were lifted and placed to kiss at the soles with my knees splayed open. I laid there in frog position, buck naked, being painted by something cold.

"We need to drip the medicine higher," Tony Blair explained leaning over, hovering an inch above my face. I'd just been flipped like a monkey in space so the anesthesia could seep up my torso. *A harsh punishment for trying to be funny, if you ask me.*

Twenty-eight minutes later, a baby's cry filled the room. One minute after that, another.

And then I was a mother to a beautiful and healthy baby boy and baby girl. *My precious Jack. My beloved Annie.*

And now, I know. . .

I know they stitched me up afterward. I see the scar. I remember feeling them sewing—in, out, yank, tug, pull, in, *OY!*—while reciting in my head the nursery rhyme:

All the King's Horses
And all the King's Men
Couldn't put Humpty together again.

But I cannot be put back together again.

As F. Scott Fitzgerald has this powerful line, "I left my capacity for hoping on the little roads that led to Zelda's sanitarium," I left something on my walk down the fluorescent-lit hallway that led to the delivery room, wheeling an IV in one hand, holding a hospital gown closed with the other. Maybe for imagining a time when I did not know you. Love you. Smell you. Constantly worry about you. Look into your deep-blue eyes. Curl your impossibly tiny fingers around each of my pinkies—it is all I ever wanted to do. (I look like a giant compared to you.) I kiss your soft little heads when you cry, and whisper, *shh, I got you, babies, I got you.*

People say there is nothing like holding your child in your arms for the first time. Of all the things people will tell you in life, I believe this will be the most true. It is so intense; so peaceful. So strange; so beautiful. So humbling; so empowering. So primal; so divine. So complicated; so simple. So clear; so confusing. And somewhere in the dizzying mist of all this paradox, is perfection. Proof that life is bigger than us. Proof that there are things that words cannot describe.

A lot has happened this past month.

I have been pooped and peed on no less than one hundred and fifty-seven (157) times, and sprayed with my own breast milk like a rap star's girlfriend in a music video getting gratuitously hosed in slow motion with champagne.

I have mastered the art of eating while walking, talking, and doing anything and everything on the go at the same time.

I have perfected the double feeding: One of you on each knee, or on each Boppy pillow, in a bouncer seat, on each side of my giant nursing pillow, "my Twin Brest Friend."

(I love you, Twin Brest Friend.)

I have touched my toes, worn shoes that tied, dropped the soap in the shower and picked it up, and held in my pee just because I could.

I have been utterly flabbergasted by the ability of my own voice to reach such high octaves, especially in the morning when I miss you already after a mere three-hour span.—"HI, angel bay-BEES! Good MORN-ing!"—

I have cried. A lot. At least once a day, often brought on by music. I bet Bob Marley never dreamed the tears that could fall while the words "every little thing is gonna be all right" is being sung. In fact, I may have to ban the Jack Johnson station on Pandora in case that "Somewhere Over the Rainbow" song comes on in order to get through the day without having to explain, "Sorry, babies, Mommy isn't sad, Mommy is crying because she's happy. She's so very, very happy."

(I'm so happy, my heart might burst.)

I have also cried the two (2) times I went out without you because I missed you. The first time I was as far as the driveway on my way to Home Depot to buy you guys a mini-fridge for your room. (Pretty soon the house will have a double set of everything. I will not be had by stairs.)

(Oh, and I noted that if you are single the best place to meet guys would be at a Home Depot 4:30 on a Tuesday afternoon for the male-to-female ratio alone.)

I have completely disconnected from society not watching the news or reading the newspaper but instead watching only the shows that Nanny, who is here to help us, has on: *General Hospital*, *The View*, *Dancing With the Stars*, *Oprah*, made-for-television holiday movies on the Hallmark Channel, or the Food Network. I have watched Rachel Ray make chicken schnitzel, twice.

I looked at your father and realized that I love him now even more, if that is even possible. . .

Oh, it's been a month, babies.

My sweet little Annie, you love throwing your hands up high in the air and dropping your chin to your chest as if you are on the Scream Machine at Great Adventure. You do this often, in the car, during burping, stretching out on the couch on your Boppy. I can't help but look at you and think that you are telling me, *Mom, enjoy the ride. . .*

And you, my gentle little Jack, you turn into a red-faced screaming pumpkin during diaper changes. Is it the cold? The nakedness? The fact that you just peed yourself innately infringing upon your manhood? Regardless, you *hate* getting your diaper changed, and you fight. You wriggle. You worm. You bellow to the heavens, "wuh-AHHHHH!" Or sometimes, my favorite, you open your mouth so wide to build up to a scream but out comes no sound. You do everything in your tiny power to try to get me to stop. . . changing. . . that. . . diaper, when the truth is, sorry, buddy, you are never going to win. I am always going to change you. Yet, you fight. . .

I love how you guys never heard of multi-tasking. You concentrate on doing one thing at a time and you do that well. You eat. You sleep. You play. You can be still. You are so present. You actually sit and look at a wall. You don't do five million things at once. You don't fork a salad, check email on your laptop, text on your phone, flip through a catalog and unknowingly get sucked into a bad movie on TV in the background and before you know it, end up watching *Don't Mess With the Zohan.*

So to both of you on your one month birthday, I say thank you. I gave you life and give you life, providing food, shelter, love, but clearly you are showing me how to live it.

Thank you, my little Zen masters, thank you.

The second day in the hospital I was scolded by a plump lactation consultant who I imagined drank Celestial Seasonings and had a lot of cats. I tried to explain to her that I was not crazy about her proposed two-hour feeding plan, which would require breast-feeding each of you individually, then giving you formula from a bottle to ensure you were getting enough food, then sitting down with the flux-capacitor-breast-pump for about twenty-five minutes to help boost up my milk supply to sustain two hungry babies who at birth weighed 6'13" and 6'3". Forget cup size. I am inflated beyond alphabet proportions, approaching a float for *Hustler* in the Thanksgiving Day parade. Your father looks at my body horrifyingly from afar. *"You're like Wonder Woman. . ."*

"But, if they eat every two to three hours, and it takes me two hours to do a feeding, aren't I always going to be feeding?"

"This is your job now," she answered abruptly. "This is not the time to party."

I blinked at her. *And your job is what, lactation consultant? Is this something you always wanted to be? Did you always have an intense fondness for breast milk?*

I considered my surreal setting.

The IV in my wrist.

The catheter dangling from beneath the sheets.

My ass-less gown.

The champagne cork rolling around on the floor from when everyone had gathered to toast your arrival as I threw up in a bedpan, a side effect from the anesthesia.

The cocktail napkins Mimi had brought that said, "The time to be happy is now, the place to be happy is here. . ."

I looked at you, my two beautiful babies sleeping peacefully in the corner.

And I thought, *screw you, lady. The party has just begun.*

Hello, My Name is Mom

Thursday, August 4, 2011

   . . . And then the couple walks in.

   They take seats across from each other at a table nestled in the back.

   What would I say if seated across from a stranger right now?

   I would say, *I know a story about the meaning of life.*

   And I know exactly where I would begin.

I Love You Forever,
Mom.

Amy Denby is a former entertainment editor for Seventeen and More magazines where she wrote book and movie reviews. She was also a staff copywriter and producer for J.Crew. For more of her writing and updates on crazy life, please visit her Web site, www.amydenby.com.

www.ingramcontent.com/pod-product-compliance
Lightning Source LLC
Chambersburg PA
CBHW050435290526
45786CB00006B/2035